T0197619

FACES & BRACES
DR WILLIAM CLARK

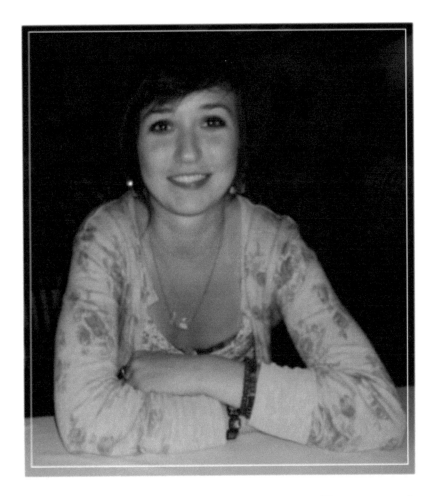

My name is Rebecca and I want to talk to you about Orthodontics For You & Me

Treat Yourself to a Brilliant Smile!

AuthorHouse™ UK
1663 Liberty Drive
Bloomington, IN 47403 USA
www.authorhouse.co.uk
Phone: 0800 047 8203 (Domestic TFN)
+44 1908 723714 (International)

Because of the dynamic nature of the Internet, any web addresses or links contained in this book may have changed since publication and may no longer be valid. The views expressed in this work are solely those of the author and do not necessarily reflect the views of the publisher, and the publisher hereby disclaims any responsibility for them.

Any people depicted in stock imagery provided by Getty Images are models, and such images are being used for illustrative purposes only.
Certain stock imagery © Getty Images.

This book is printed on acid-free paper.

ISBN: 978-1-7283-5219-0 (sc)
ISBN: 978-1-7283-5218-3 (e)

Library of Congress Control Number: 2020906956

Print information available on the last page.

Published by AuthorHouse 05/06/2020

authorHOUSE

FACES & BRACES

DR WILLIAM CLARK

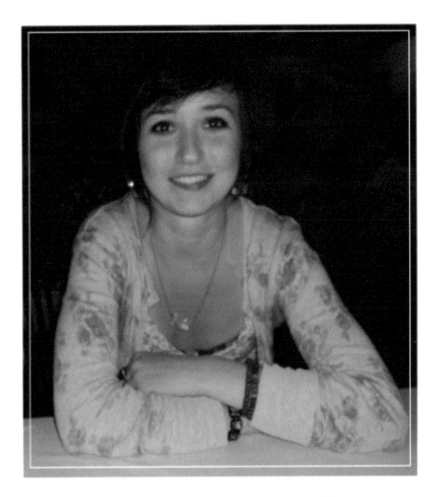

My name is Rebecca and I want to talk to you about
Orthodontics For You & Me

Treat Yourself to a Brilliant Smile!

A file of New Horizons in Orthodontics Limited

© 2012 New Horizons in Orthodontics Limited

http://www.newhorizonsinorthodontics.com

http://www.twinblocks.com

The right of William J.Clark identified as author of this work has been asserted by him in accordance with the Copyright, Designs and Patents Act, 1998

First Edition© 2012
ISBN 978-0-9570929-1-4

Note:

Medical knowledge is constantly changing. As new information becomes available, changes in treatment, procedures, equipment and the use of materials becomes necessary. The author and publishers have taken care to ensure that the information given in this text is acccurate and up to date. However, readers are strongly advised to confirm that the information, especially with regard to materials for intra-oral use complies with the latest legislation and standards of practice.

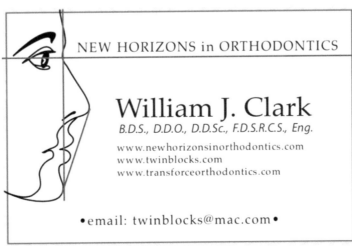

NEW HORIZONS in ORTHODONTICS

William J. Clark
B.D.S., D.D.O., D.D.Sc., F.D.S.R.C.S., Eng.
www.newhorizonsinorthodontics.com
www.twinblocks.com
www.transforceorthodontics.com

• email: twinblocks@mac.com •

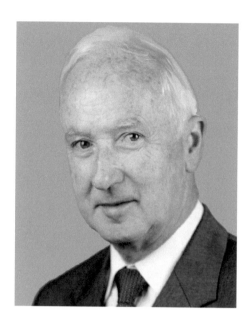

About the Author

Dr Clark has 50 years experience in orthodontic practice and continues to develop innovative appliances in orthodontic and orthopaedic techniques. In 1977 he developed Twin Blocks in his orthodontic practice in Scotland and has taught Twin Block Technique worldwide.

In 2004 he designed TransForce Lingual appliances for arch development with support from Ortho Organizers, and has recently developed Fixed Twin Blocks as a new advance in functional therapy

Dr Clark is the first recipient of an award of distinction from the British Orthodontic Society for an outstanding contribution to the specialty of orthodontics. In 2008 he received an award from the International Functional Association for personal outstanding international service to functionalism and orthodontics.

New e-books, 'Advances in Fixed Appliance Technique' and 'Advances in Functional Therapy & Dentofacial Orthopaedics' provide a comprehensive account of fixed and functional appliance therapy.

Further information is available on www.twinblocks.com

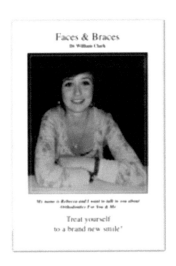

"This book on patient education is outstanding"
Dr Ramesh Sabhlok (B.D.S., M.D.S., M. Orth RCS (Eng)

"The book is written in an informal style that will be easy to read and understand for both teenagers and adults alike. There are sections including humorous dialogues and questions and answers, making it both a fun and informative read. It would be a useful addition to any orthodontic office and I would enthusiastically recommend it to parents and patients, both young and old."

Amy Meng Lei B.D.S., Kings College University, London

"I really enjoyed the message and how it was delivered from the patient's perspective by someone of their same age group."

Professor Emeritus Katherine Vig, Ohio State University.

This is a very fine example of how fantastic eBooks are.
I had the experience of reviewing this eBook on the iPad, and it really fits well on this platform. The cost is pretty affordable and attractive, and I believe this can be a nice contribution for both patient education and marketing strategy.

Professor Jorge Faber,
Editor in Chief
Journal of the World Federation of Orthodontics

The chatty style of writing coming from Rebecca and her interaction with some of the subjects comes over as very realistic. The text is encouraging and engaging. The photography is particularly good and 'clean' giving the impression that the photos were taken in a setting of care and responsibility"

Eldon Zuill,
Manager of Health Education Board of Scotland

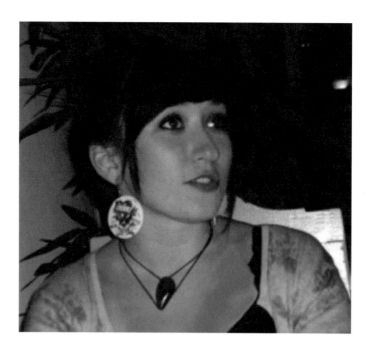

Rebecca wants to talk to you about Faces & Braces

Would you like to improve your image and your prospects in life?
This book can change your life!
Whether you're a youngster, a teenager, or an adult
If you are embarrassed to smile because of your teeth
'Faces & Braces' will help you to smile with confidence..
Do you have crooked teeth?
Do your front teeth stick out?
Does your chin stick out?
Do you lack confidence?
This book has answers for these problems.
Catch up on Cool Chat !
Did you know that the Tin Grin is the In Thing?
Train Tracks are Trendy!
Brace yourself for a Brilliant Smile!
Would you like 'train tracks' or invisible braces?
Gary was teased at school until he fought back in the gym.
His teeth don't stick out any more and now he's the team captain
Are you anxious about your own smile or one of your family?
Read on to see what happened to Gary and his friends
This is the best investment you will ever make in your self image!

ORTHODONTICS
FOR YOU & ME

Topics:

I have a gap between my front teeth!

Fixed Or Removable Braces?

Rebecca Meets Gary   Faces & Braces

In the Boys Gym .... Gary Fights Back !

I don't show my upper teeth when I smile

My chin sticks out too much!

What are Functional Appliances?

Twin Blocks Improved My Face

Why are Braces called Train Tracks?

Train Tracks Are Trendy !

Cool Chat .... In the Girls Cloakroom

Your treatment depends on the shape of your face

Bracket Design

Adults Prefer Aesthetic Appliances

Tony's invisible braces

My teeth are straight. Why do I have to wear Retainers?

Braces Are Cool !

Orthodontics Can Change Your Life

Teeth are for eating!

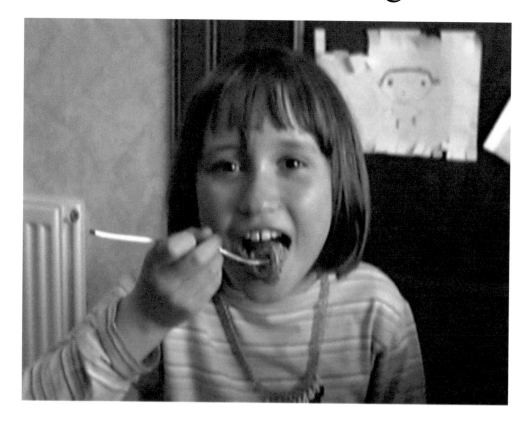

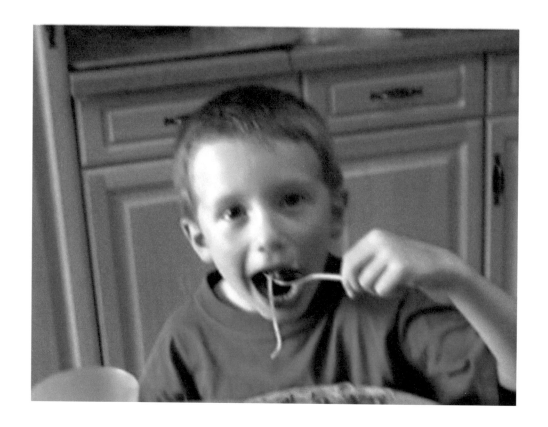

Teeth show you are HAPPY!

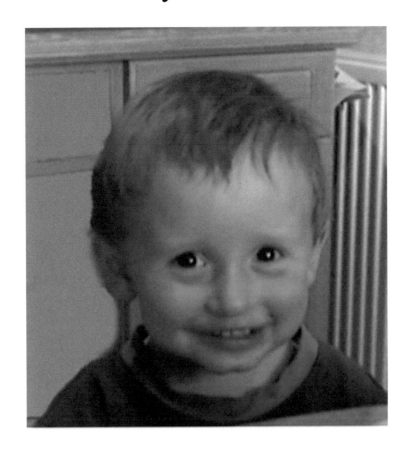

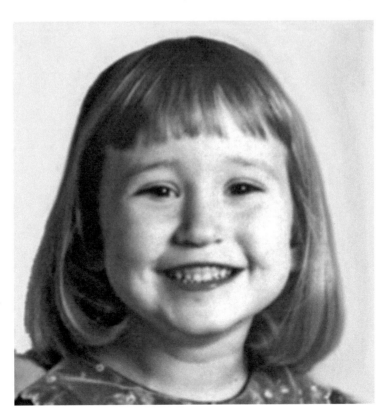

Teeth are for smiling !

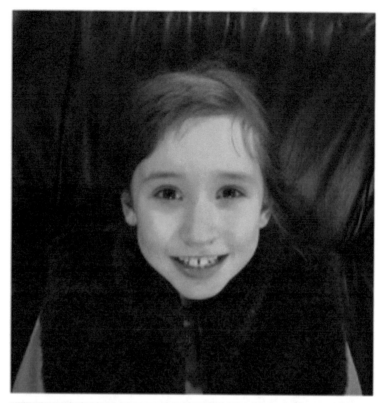

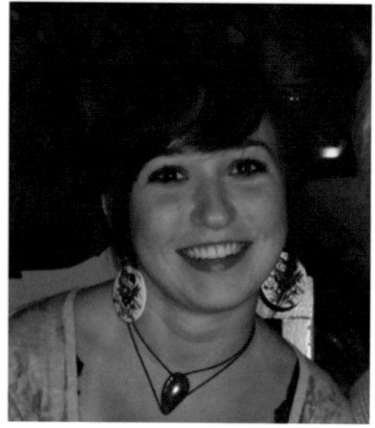

This is me when I was 8

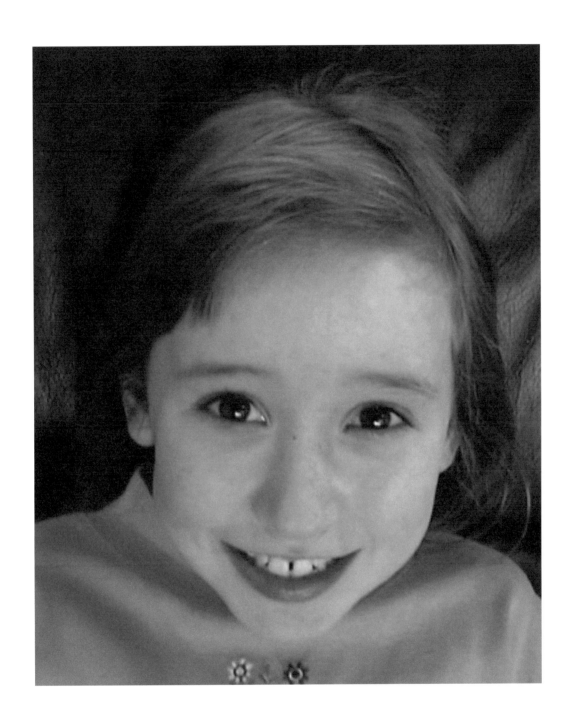

I have a gap between my front teeth!

I had treatment when I was eight!

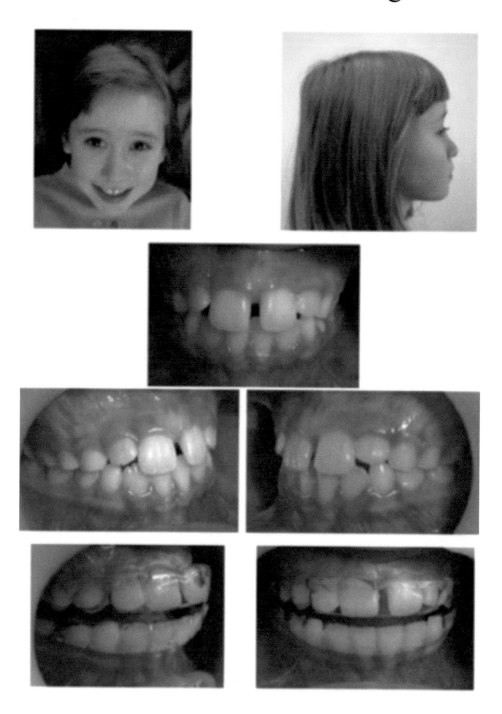

Don't worry if you have a small gap between your upper front teeth at my age. I had an appliance like a gum shield that I wore every night. You wear it when you watch television or play a computer game.

That was the only treatment I needed!

I'm so glad I had my teeth fixed when I was young!

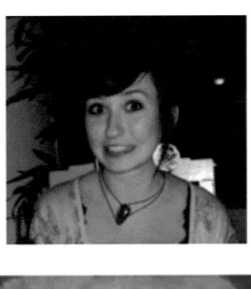

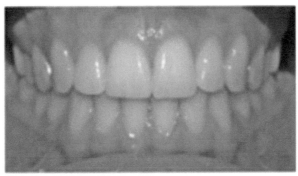

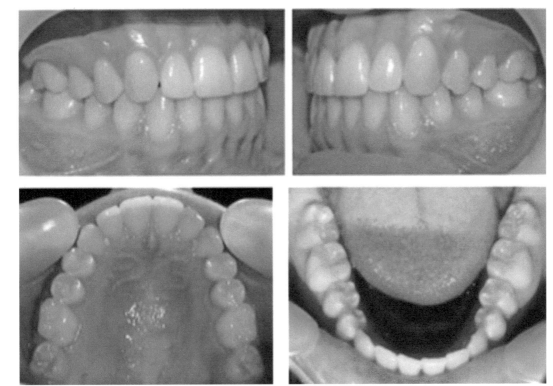

Q: What are removable appliances?

A: They are sometimesused for early treatment
This appliance has a screw to expand the upper arch
This helps to correct the front teeth for a young patient
We can use these before the patient is ready for Train Tracks

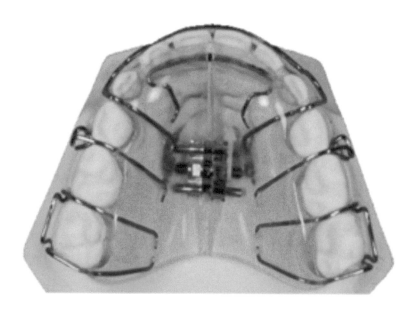

Removable appliances don't work in your pocket!
Your treatment will fail if you don't wear them all the time

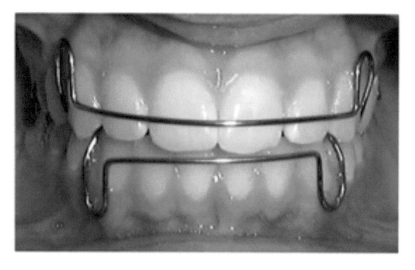

These are removable retainers

They prevent the teeth from moving after treatment

Anterior Teeth

4 Incisors & 2 Canines

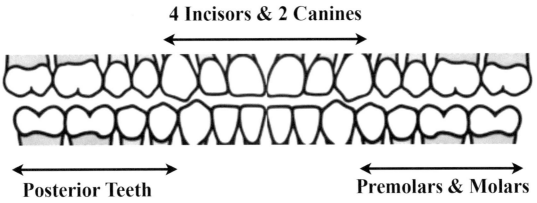

Posterior Teeth

Premolars & Molars

Upper Arch: Maxilla

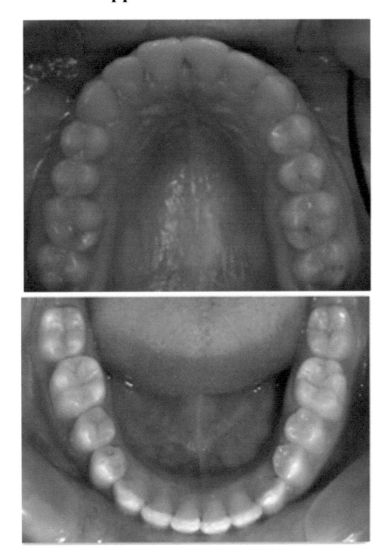

Lower Arch: Mandible

Perfect Archform

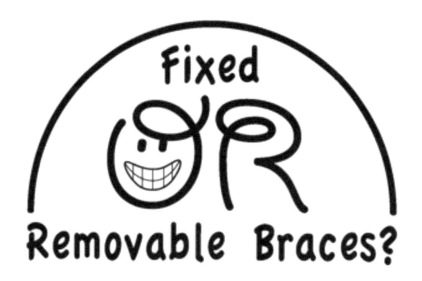

**Q: My teeth are crooked and I don't like my smile.
Do I need fixed or removable braces?**

**A: When teeth are crooked or do not bite correctly
There is a malocclusion**

Treatment depends on what the problem is
We have to decide if it is just your teeth
Or is it related to the size of your jaws?
Your upper front teeth may stick out
Because you have a small lower jaw
Or your lower jaw may be too big
Functional appliances correct the jaw position
Orthopaedic appliances treat severe problems
Removable appliances help in early treatment
But you may need a fixed appliance later
Removable and Fixed Appliances treat different problems

REBECCA MEETS GARY

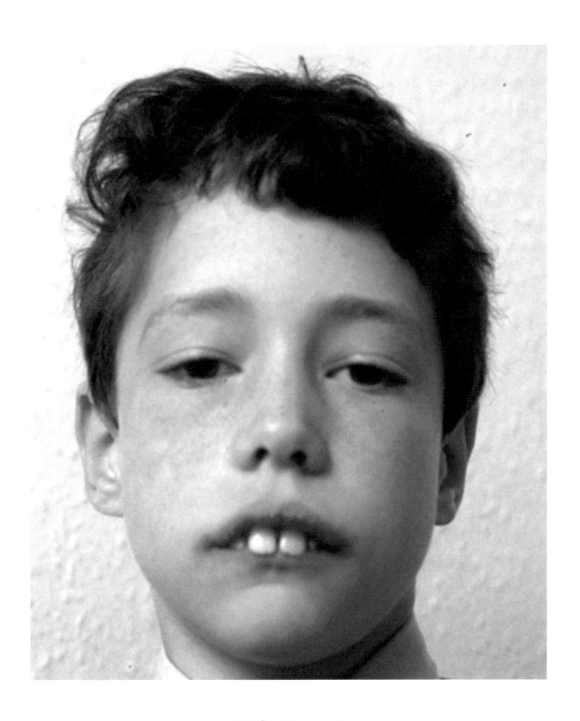

Hi Gary!
I want to talk to you about
Faces & Braces

Faces and Braces

R: Have you seen this new book, about 'Faces and Braces'

G: What do Faces have to do with Braces?
I use braces to hold up my trousers
(Some people call them suspenders)

R: Not that kind of braces, the kind that fix your teeth

G: Oh, you mean Train Tracks

R: Train Tracks are not the only kind of braces in orthodontics

G: What is Orthodontics and what does that have to do with me?

R: Orthodontics means 'Straight Teeth'

G   Why should I read this book? My teeth are not straight.

R: That's exactly why you should read it.
Are you happy with your teeth?

G: All my friends tease me 'cos my teeth are crooked and stick out.

R: You could wear braces that fix your crooked teeth and your face.
That's why we're talking about 'Faces and Braces'

G: I have no confidence 'cos I'm ashamed of my teeth
They're the only teeth I have and I'm stuck with them!
Nobody could fix my face, I just don't have a chin.

R: No kidding Gary, braces could give you a chin
You could be a heart throb if you had your teeth fixed
Just look at the pictures in this book and you will understand

G: Maybe I should read it and decide for myself.

R: I think you could become a real good looking guy if you had
your teeth fixed.

Don't be shy. Just read on and go for it.

Hey Gary! How Goes It?

I'm really depressed today I have to go to the orthodontist tomorrow and he's gonna fit some gadget called a Twin Block. You can't imagine how bad I feel. It's just gonna be the worst day of my life!

Get real Gary. Do you really want your teeth to stick out for the rest of your life? The Twin Block is a fantastic deal. The Captain of the school team had Twin Blocks when he was your age and now he's a real heart throb and has to beat off the girls! What it does for you is it gives you a strong chin like a real man. No hard feelings Gary, but you really need a chin. If you want to look good when you grow up you better have TWIN BLOCKS. Go for it Gary you'll never regret it!

Hey that's what Rebecca told me. Maybe I should go and read that book she showed me! This TWIN BLOCK deal sounds like what I need.

When Gary reads the book he decides to go for it and FIGHT BACK!

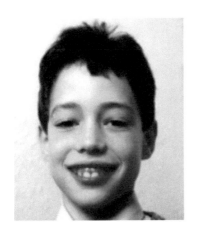 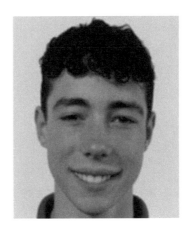

His teeth don't stick out any more and now he is the Team Captain!
Of course he is very popular with the girls !!!

Read on to see what happened to Gary

I was teased at school about my teeth
But after I spoke to Rebecca
I wore Twin Blocks to fix my face!

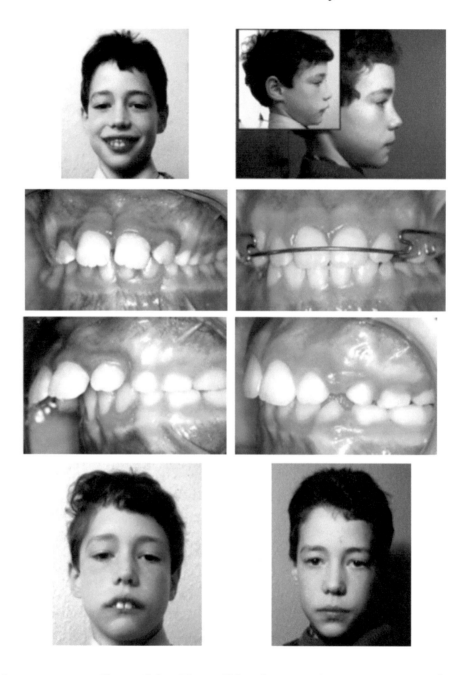

If you have a receding chin *Twin Blocks can* improve your face. Gary wore *Twin Blocks* for 8 months to guide his jaw and tongue forward. His teeth no longer stick outside his lips and he can breathe more easily.

Then I only needed Train Tracks for a short time

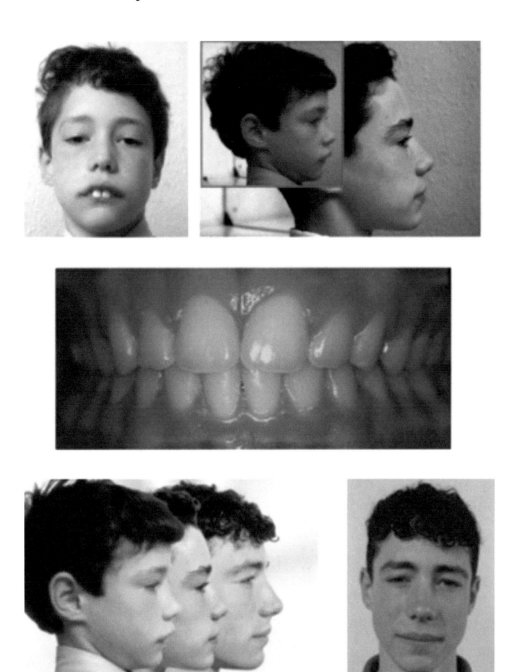

My teeth don't stick out any more!

Now I have a strong profile and a confident smile. What a great deal!
Twin Blocks fixed my face and Train Tracks fixed my smile!
Faces & Braces really work!

Malocclusions Are Inherited

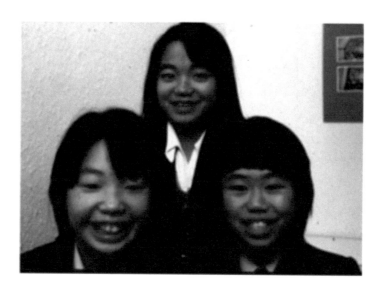

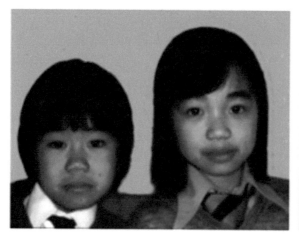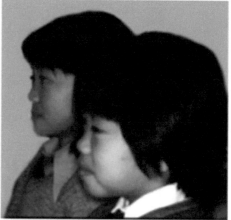

Malocclusions run in families, and we often treat brothers and sisters. Children may inherit their facial characteristics from either parent so they may not have the same features. A prominent chin may be due to a large lower jaw or a small upper jaw.

My lower teeth bite in front of my upper teeth
I don't show my upper teeth when I smile

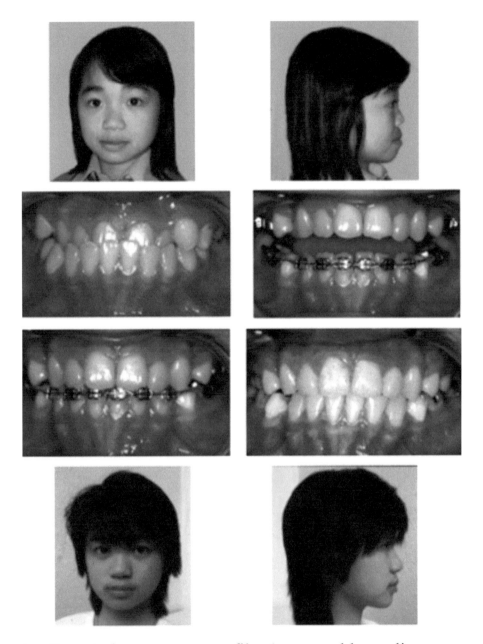

I had extractions to improve my profile. A removable appliance moved my upper teeth forward and a fixed appliance moved my lower teeth back.

It was worth it because it improved my face and corrected my bite

I wanted the same treatment as my sister!

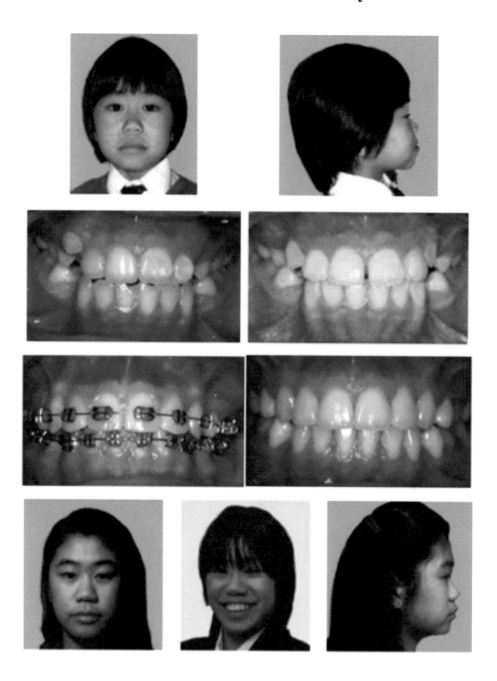

I wore a removable appliance to move my upper teeth forward.
I had extractions to move my lower teeth back to improve my
profile. Then I had Train Tracks to improve my smile.

I'm so happy that I had orthodontic treatment.

I was teased at school because my chin stuck out
Now I'm not embarrassed when I smile!

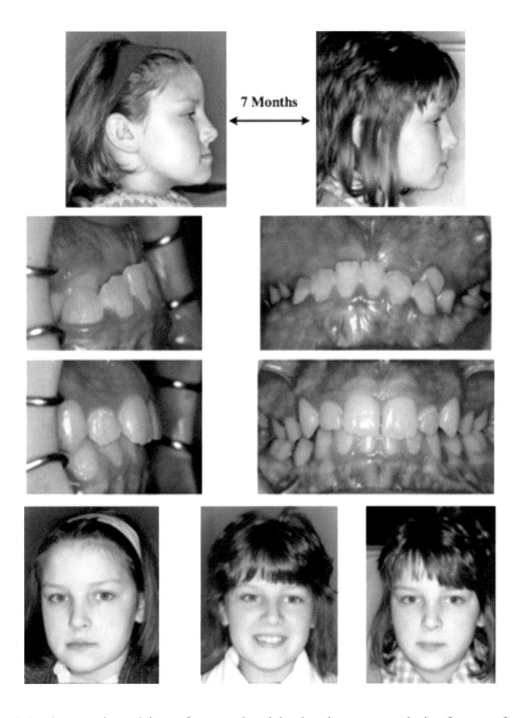

My lower jaw bites forward with the lower teeth in front of the upper teeth, Upper removable and lower fixed appliances corrected my crossbite and improved my deep bite.

When I smiled I only showed my lower teeth
Until I had Reverse Twin Blocks to correct my bite

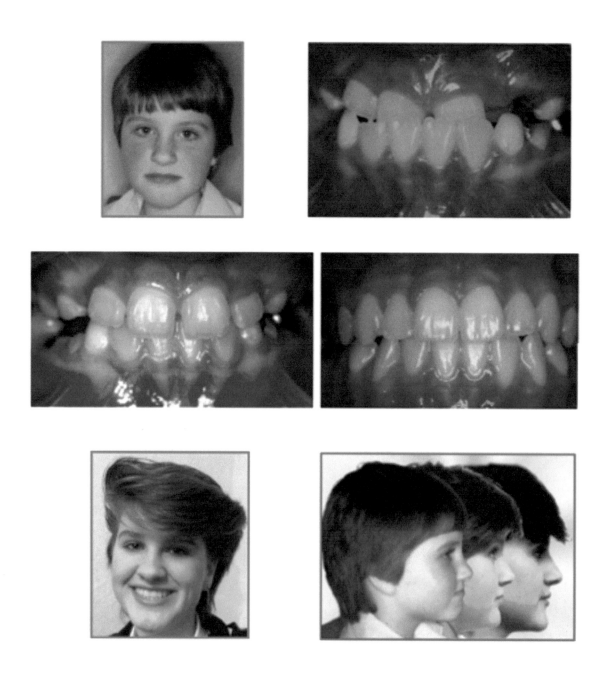

When I was 7 years old I had a a small upper jaw with my upper teeth biting behind my lower teeth. My bite was corrected after 8 months.

I didn't need any more treatment and this is me 7 years later!

MONOBLOC (1902)

The monobloc was designed for patients with a receding chin to wear at night to move the lower jaw forward to help patients to breathe better.

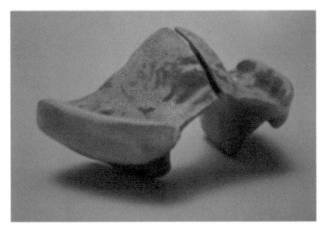

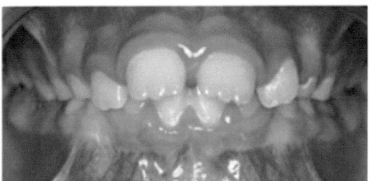

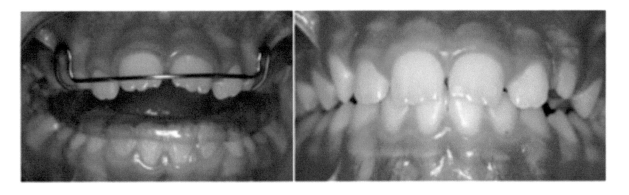

BIONATOR (1960's)

The Bionator is an updated version of the monobloc to correct the teeth and advance the lower jaw. This may also help patients to breathe better.

I was treated with a Bionator

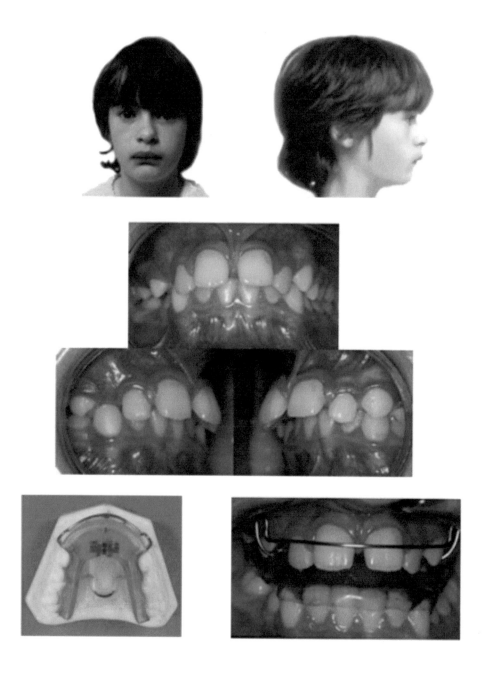

The Bionator is worn at night and when possible during the day. It interferes with speech and cannot be worn for eating.

The Bionator improved my face and my teeth

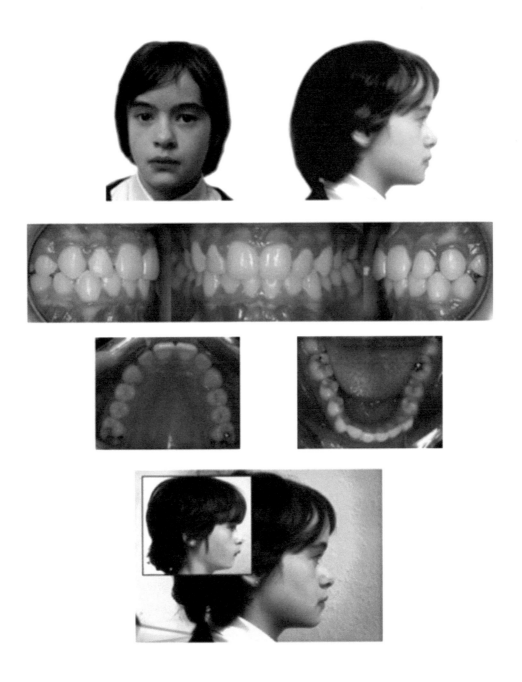

In suitable cases the Bionator produces impressive results

Q: How do you improve the face?
What are functional appliances?
A: Let's look at two typical patients

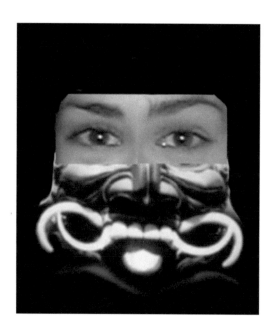

Digital Image by W. Clark 2020

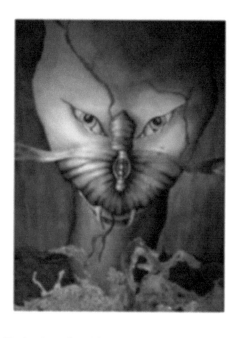

Painting by Alastair Clark 1983

Orthodontics improves the teeth

There is no way we can fit all of these teeth in this mouth. This is definitely an **orthodontic** case! This patient needs extractions, followed by braces to fix his teeth. As you can see, his face is perfectly normal!

Orthopaedics improves the face!

This is an unusual face. This is definitely an **orthopaedic** case. The teeth are no big deal, but to treat this patient we must treat the face, not just the teeth. This patient requires a functional appliance to fix his face.

Functional Appliances

Functional appliances have been used for over a hundred years to treat patients who have a small lower jaw and a receding chin. This can also help patients who suffer from sleep apnoea, and have difficulty in breathing when they are asleep.

TWIN BLOCKS

Sometimes the upper teeth seem to be prominent but the real cause is that the lower jaw is small. *Twin Blocks* are upper and lower appliances with blocks meeting on an inclined plane over the posterior teeth to guide the lower jaw forward. This improves the face and the profile for a patient who has a weak or receding chin.

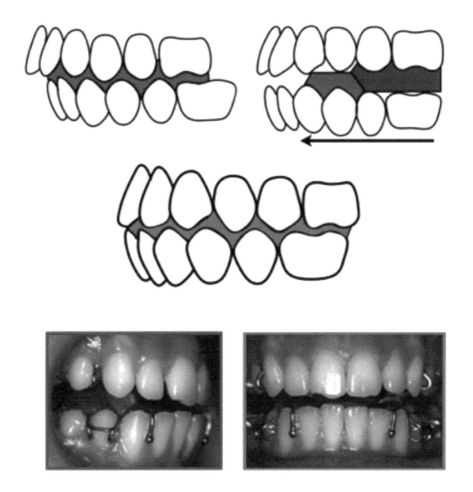

Twin Blocks are aesthetic functional appliances.
Separate upper and lower blocks guide the lower jaw forward.
Twin Blocks are comfortable to wear for eating and speaking.

Twin Blocks Improved My Face!

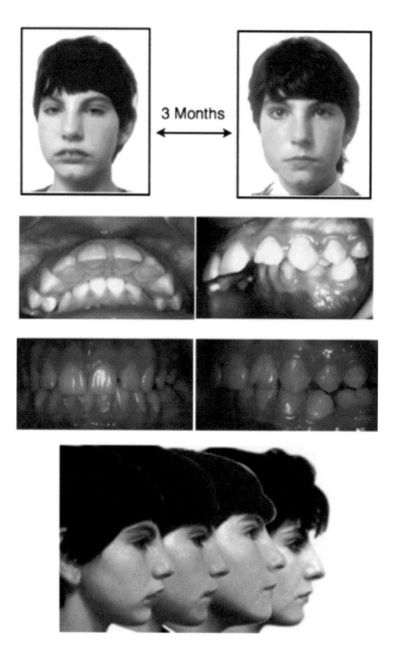

3 Months

Before Treatment: 3 Months: 11 Months: 5 Years

This girl has prominent upper teeth and a receding chin.
After 3 months treatment she looks like a different person.
Twin Blocks can fix your face and your teeth!

Predicting Facial Change
Close your teeth together
Then bite forward & close your lips

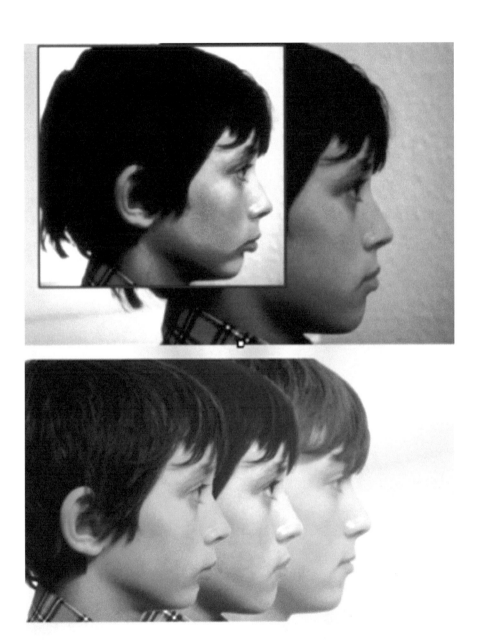

Before Treatment: Biting Forward: 11 Months Later

If your profile and face improves when you bite forward and close your lips together you may need a functional appliance.

What You See Is What You Get!

Planning Functional Therapy

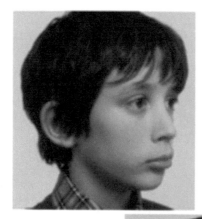

Before Treatment

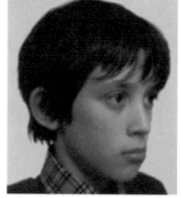

Bite Forward

Close Your Lips

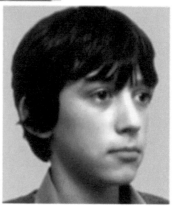

After 11 months your
face has improved

Photographs help to plan treatment with functional appliances. If your face looks better when you bite forward and close your lips you may benefit from functional therapy, but if this makes you look worse then other methods of treatment will be better for your face.

Both my face and my teeth improved
After 11 months treatment with Twin Blocks!

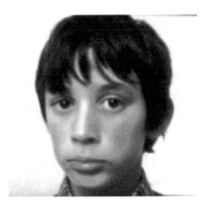 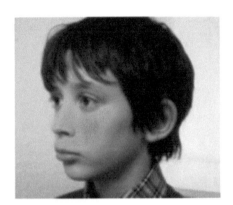

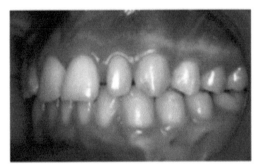

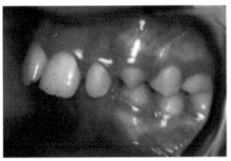

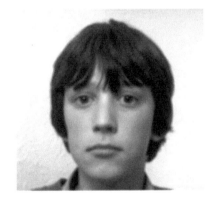 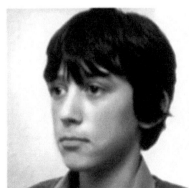

I had early treatment with Twin Blocks

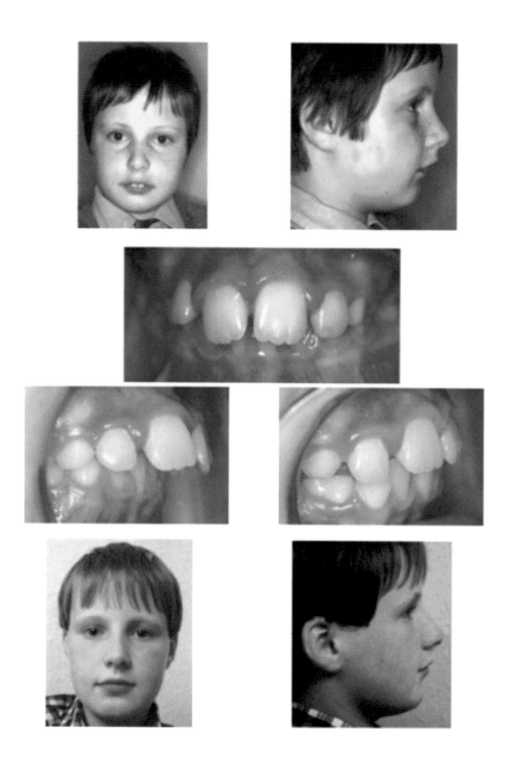

I was treated with Twin Blocks when I was 9
After 8 months my face improved
Now I can close my lips comfortably over my teeth

Twin Blocks improved my profile

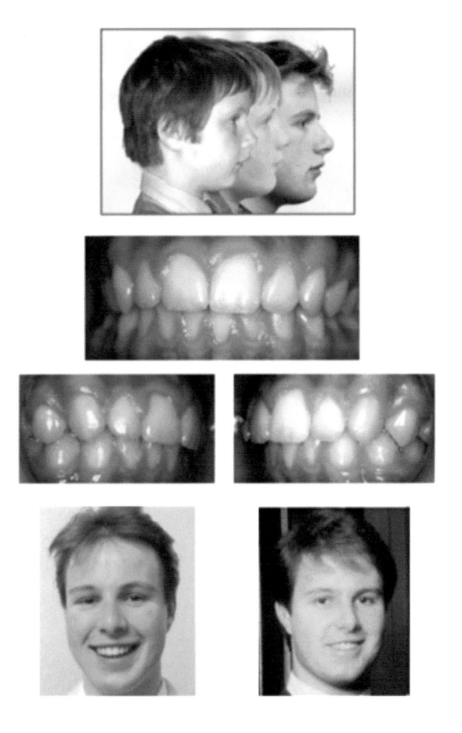

Then I didn't need Train Tracks
This helped me to mature as a young man
Now I can smile with confidence!

Twin Blocks fixed my face!

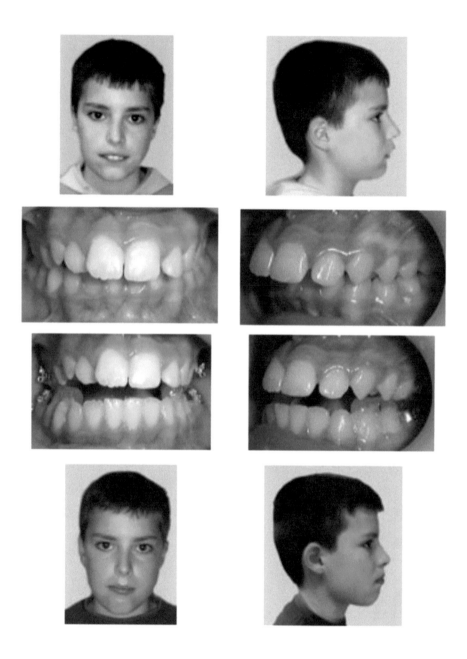

Twin Blocks guided my lower jaw forward.
My appearance improved when Twin Blocks were fitted
My lips now close comfortably over my teeth.

I have a confident smile six years later

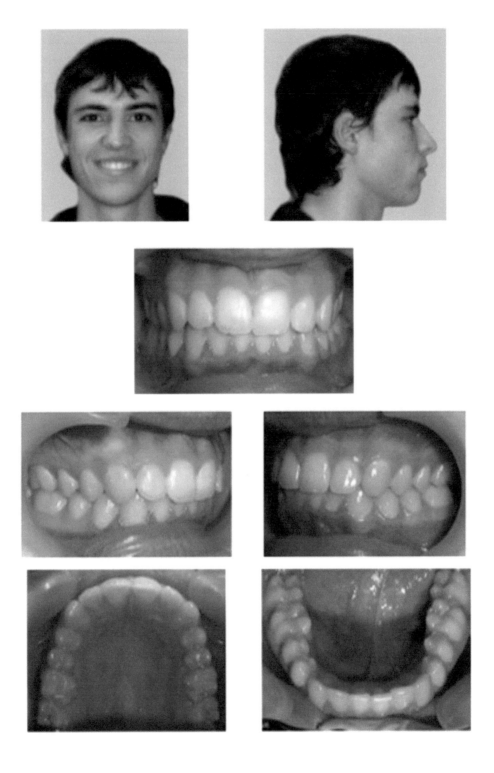

Unlike many cosmetic procedures the benefits of Twin Block functional therapy last for a lifetime.

Twin Blocks made me more confident!

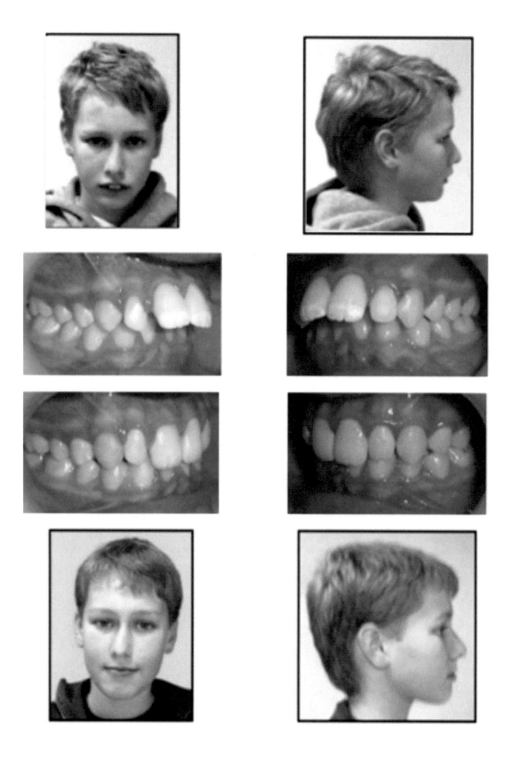

Twin Blocks improve your appearance
This improves your self image.
You gain confidence and it can transform your life.

Q: My son's teeth are prominent and he can't close his lips so he breathes through his mouth. Can you help this by moving his teeth?

A:We sometimes have to extract teeth to improve the face. In this case two upper and two lower teeth were removed and Train Tracks moved the teeth back. Now he can comfortably close his lips.

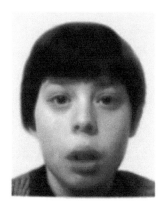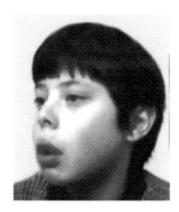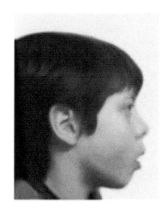

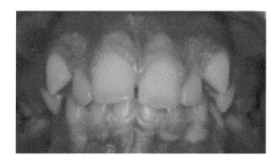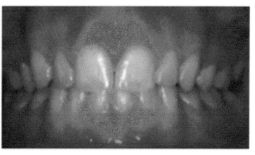

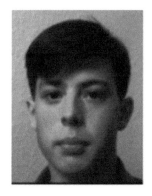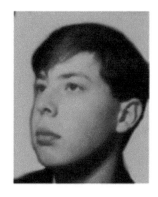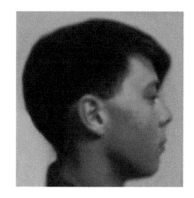

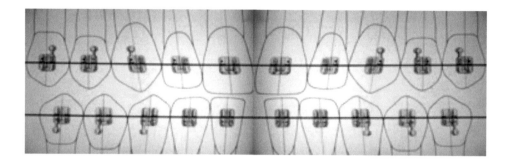

FIXED APPLIANCES place brackets on the teeth with a wire running through the brackets. Someone thought this looked like Train Tracks. The name was popular with kids so it stuck.

Q: What is a bracket?
It sounds like something you use to fix up a shelf in DIY!

There are many different designs of brackets, but they all work on the same principle. A wire runs through grooves in the brackets and is held in place with small elastic ties or a locking mechanism. Flexible wires apply gentle pressure to move the teeth. The teeth move towards the wire, which is a perfect arch form. That is what makes the teeth straight when they are tied to the wire.

The wires are changed during your treatment, starting with flexible wires and moving gradually to thicker wires that hold the teeth in position at the end of treatment.

Is it painful to wear braces?

You have some discomfort when braces are fitted and after they are adjusted. This lasts for the first day or two but soon settles down. Some patients are more sensitive then others and they may take pain killers if necessary, but this doesn't apply to most patients. You will receive instructions on cleaning your teeth and appliances and you must avoid hard and sticky foods as these will damage your appliance and make your treatment time much longer.

I have heard about invisible braces. What are they?

Some patients, especially adults prefer invisible appliances. There are several different types of invisible braces. Some are made of clear material that fits over the teeth. They are called aligners. Clear aesthetic brackets are almost invisible as they reflect the colour of the teeth.
Lingual Brackets fit behind the teeth and are used mostly in adult therapy

Invisible Appliances for Arch Development

Lingual Appliances also fit behind the teeth so they are invisible. They are designed to correct the teeth by applying pressure to the inner surfaces of the teeth. We will talk more about this later.

Diagram courtesy of Rocky Mountain Orthodontics

Elastics tie the wires into the brackets

Bright Elastics Are Fashionable for Girls

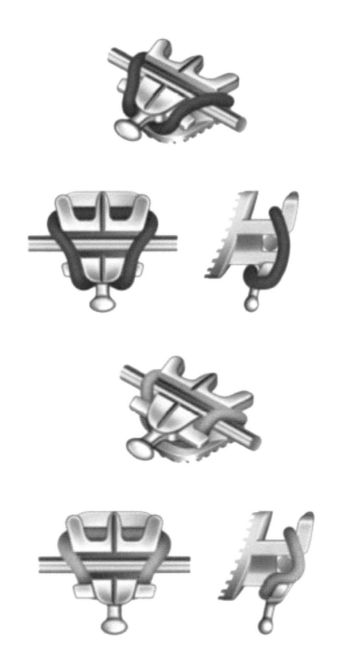

Boys often choose team colors

Self Ligating Brackets

Self Ligating Brackets open and close with a locking mechanism. It is personal preference whether you choose self ligating or elastic ties. School kids tend to have fun choosing the coloured ties.

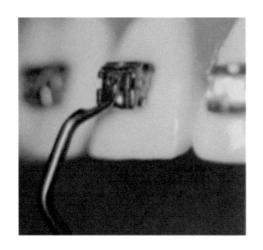 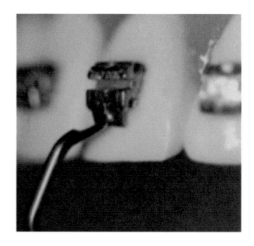

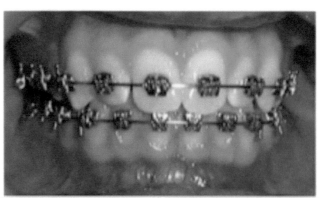

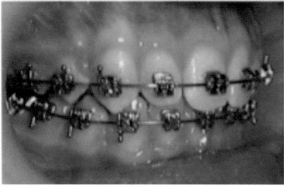 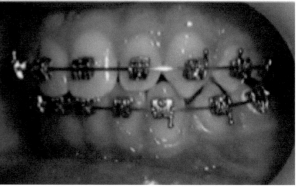

Self Ligating Brackets are easier to keep clean and some adults prefer them. However adults also like invisible appliances.

Adults Prefer Aesthetic Brackets

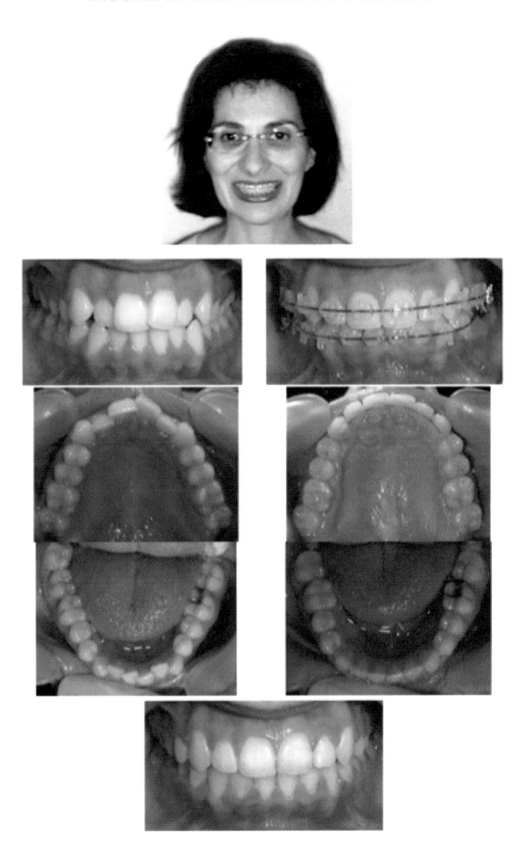

Cool Chat

In .... The Girls Cloakroom
I'm so nervous 'cos I go to the orthodontist tomorrow to get my braces.

Why on earth are you nervous? I already have mine and it's not a big deal having braces fitted. Don't worry, it's one of the biggest days in your life! Braces 'R so Cool. I look on it as a Fashion Accessory, every bit as good as bling. In fact Braces 'R the IN thing. You're kind of out of the club nowadays if you don't have braces.

But doesn't it hurt? It must be painful

Putting the braces on doesn't hurt at all. Your orthodontist will tie little wires in and that will feel a bit tight at first and it is uncomfortable for a couple of days because it is beginning to move your teeth right at the start. Then it settles down and it's O.K. Look at my colours I had them changed last week.
I went for Cool colours this time, but you can change them at every visit. It's great fun! You really have to think what you're going to be wearing and choose your colours to match. Don't be shy about it. You want to make a statement. Be proud of your braces. You get much more attention, first from your family. they probably give you treats 'cos you have braces. Then your friends are really interested and even jealous! Make the most of it.

Then of course there's the boys! That's the best bit. I never had so much attention. All of a sudden they noticed me! And I can't wait until I'm finished my treatment and have a dazzling smile. Then they really will notice me, for the rest of my life! All good!

But how does it affect your social life ?

It's a definite plus. Just think how you look in the disco! Under the lights your braces shine like diamonds. The other fun part is that I can choose my ear rings and bling to match my braces. Shiny metallic accessories go very well, like ear rings or a pendant. Then you can pick up the colours of the little elastics with your outfit.

Even at school it's COOL. It's like having a touch of <u>CLASS</u> in class!

It really brightens up your school uniform. Makes you stand out from the crowd!

Hey thanks so much. I'm really looking forward to having my braces now!

TRAIN TRACKS ARE TRENDY!!!

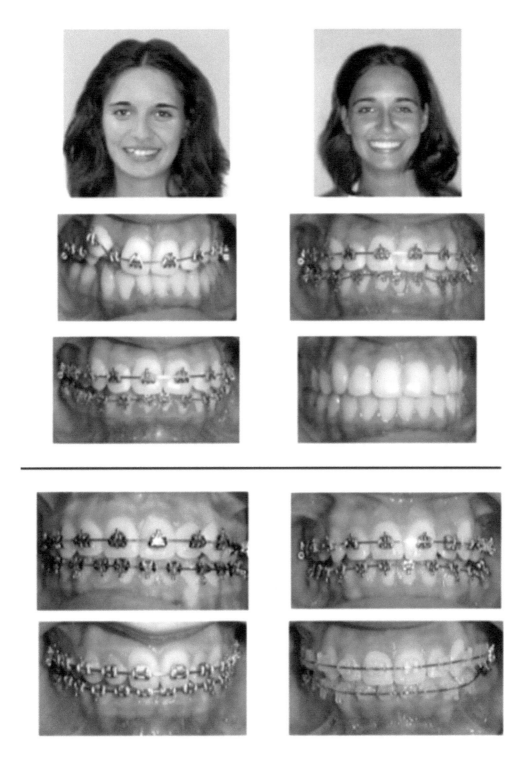

You can choose your *Train Tracks* to suit your personality.
And improve your smile at the same time

I had Train Tracks to correct my crooked teeth

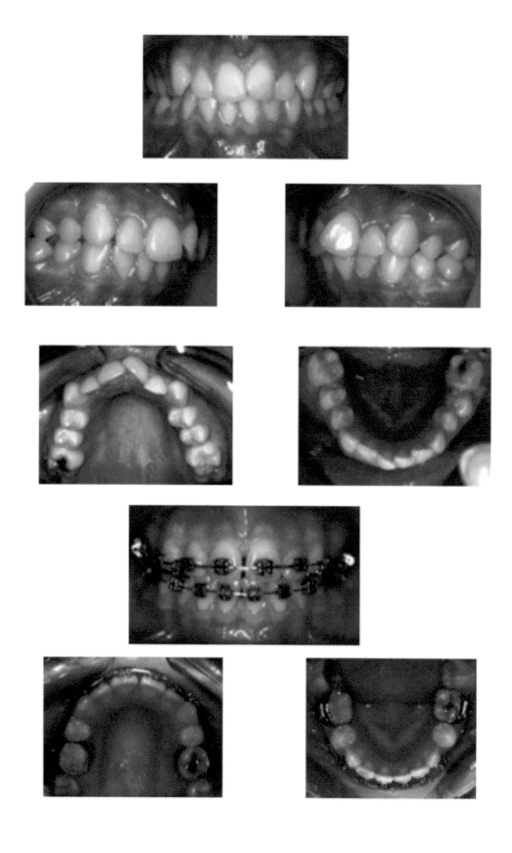

I had extractions to improve my profile

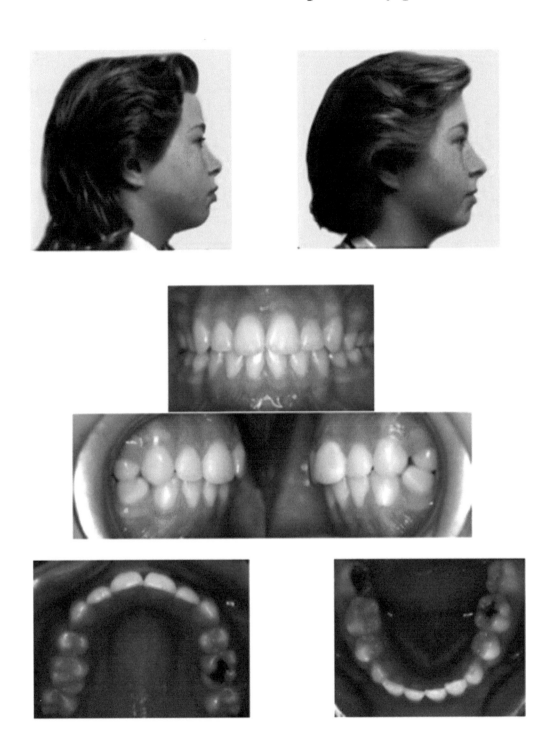

Train Tracks improved my smile and my face!

I had arch development with invisible appliances

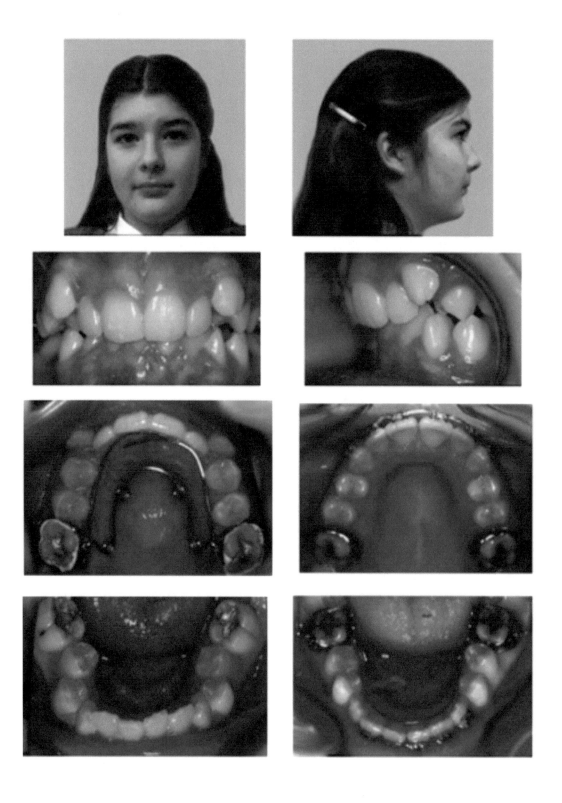

Then I had Train Tracks to complete treatment

The prize is a wide smile with perfect arch form

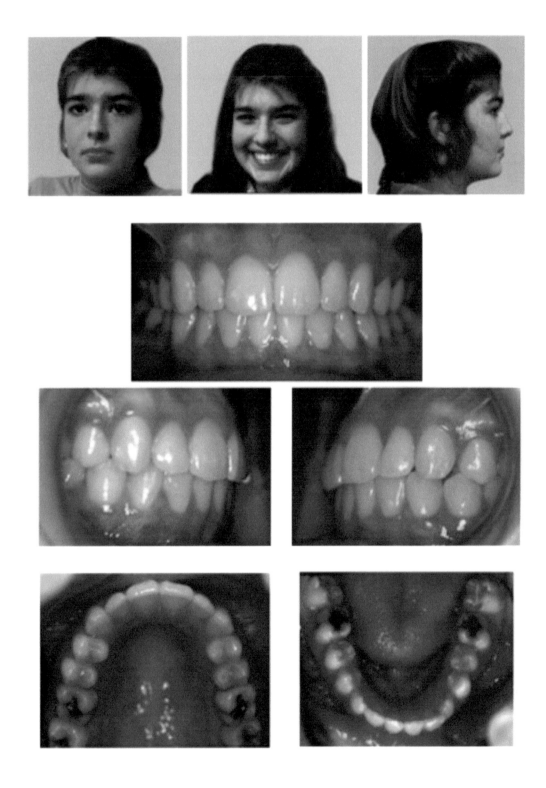

TransForce Treatment Of Dental Asymmetry

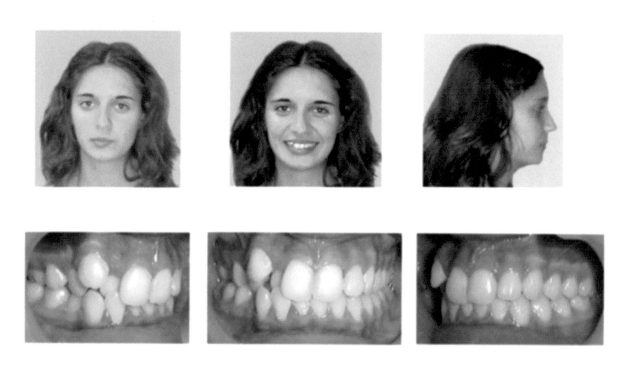

Upper Transverse Expander Corrects Arch Form

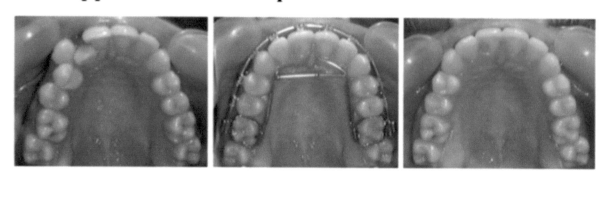

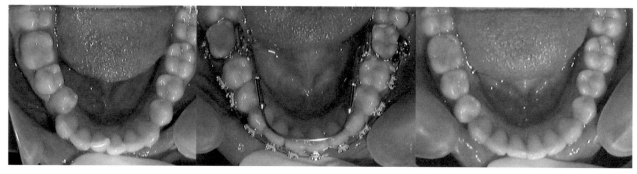

Lower Sagittal TransForce Corrects Asymmetry

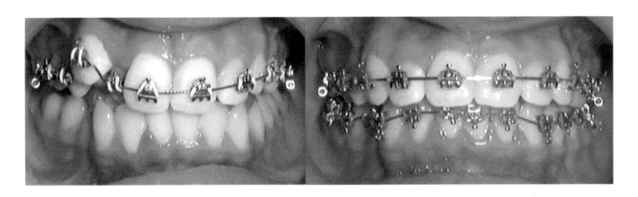

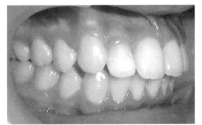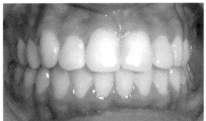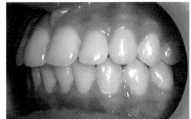

Type to enter text

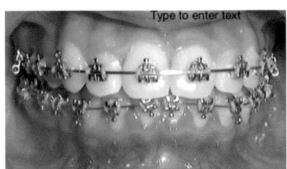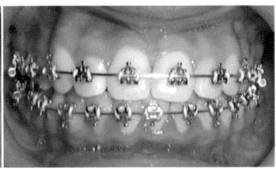

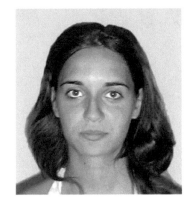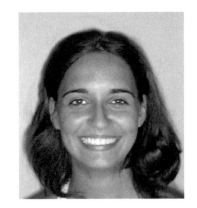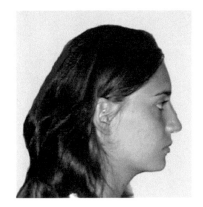

A Beautiful Smile & Improved Profile

The Prize is a Brilliant Smile

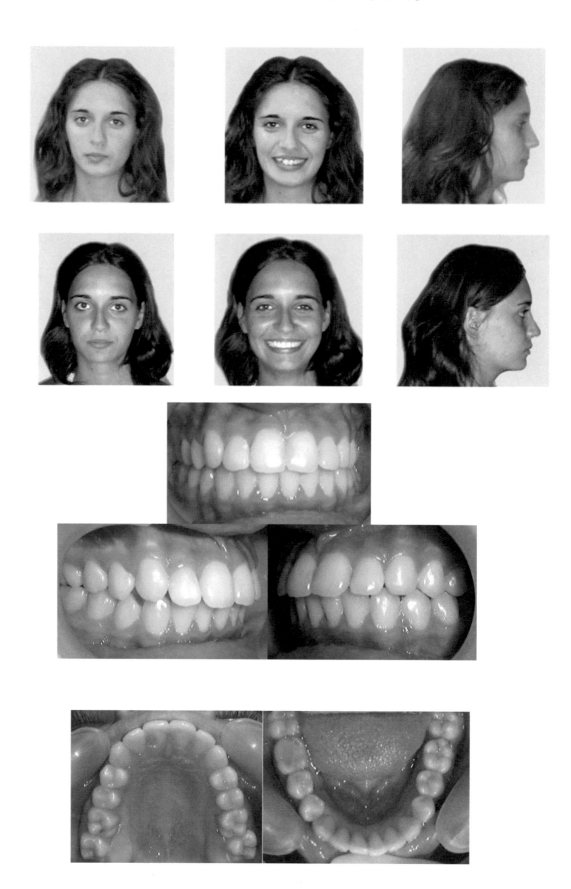

Improved Technology Shortens Treatment

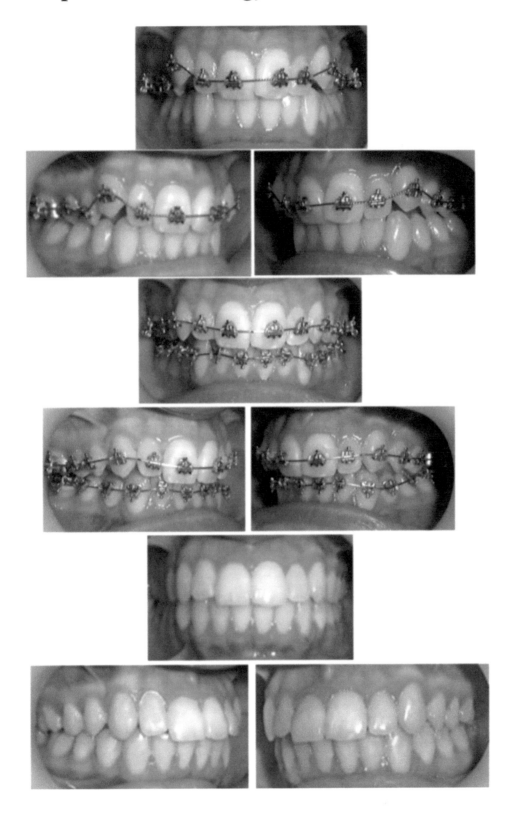

Invisible TransForce Appliances

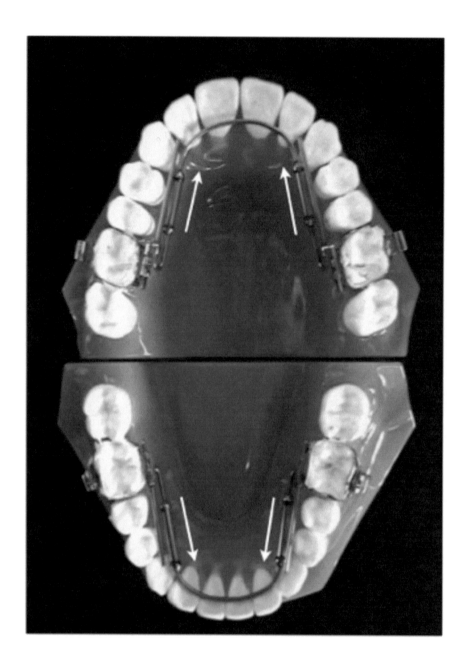

Invisible TransForce Appliances fit behind the teeth

**Springs enclosed in tubes apply gentle forces and
move the teeth more quickly than other appliances
This reduces the time in Train Tracks by 50%**

TransForce Invisible Appliances
Invisible appliances that fit behind the teeth!

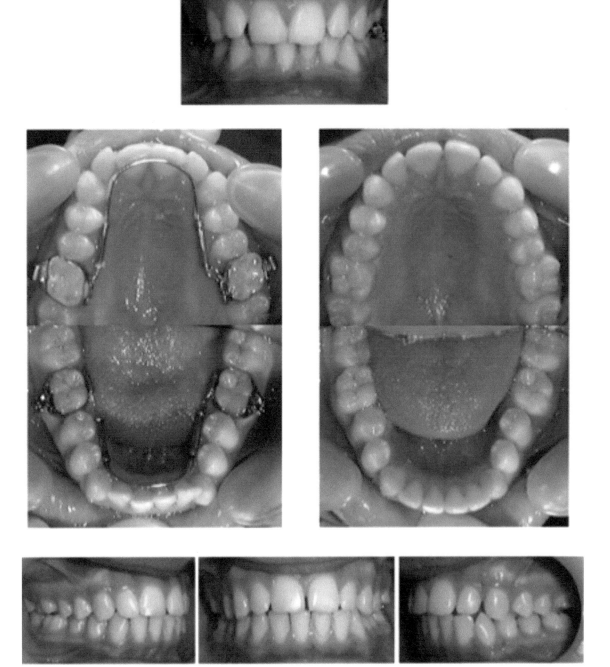

Wow! That wasn't difficult. How did you do that?
Just six months treatment!
Invisible TransForce Appliances are patient-friendly

I don't show my upper teeth when I smile because my lower teeth bite forward

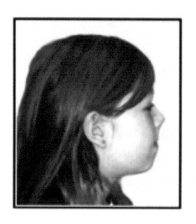 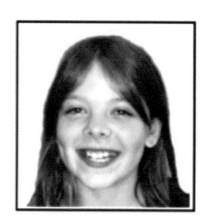

TransForce Sagittal Appliance

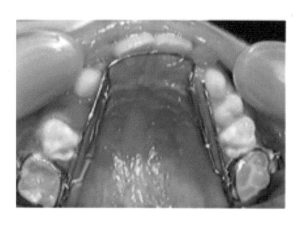 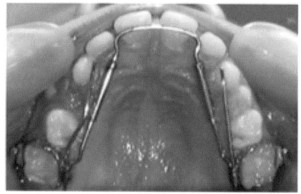

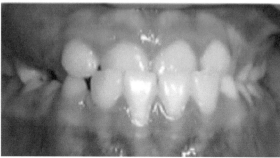 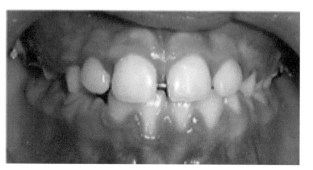

**Trendy Transforce appliances corrected my bite in 3 months
My treatment was finished in 9 months!**

This Is Me Three Years Later!

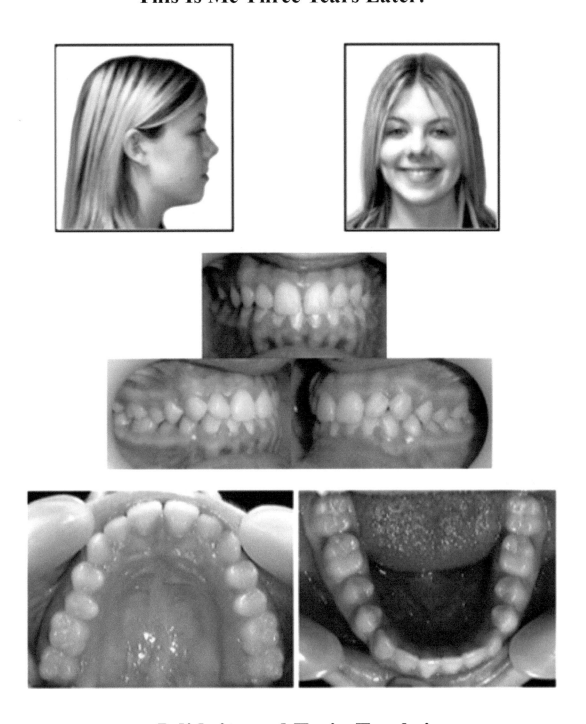

I didn't need Train Tracks!

No more treatment was needed
My profile and smile have improved
Now I can smile with confidence

TransForce ® Transverse Expander

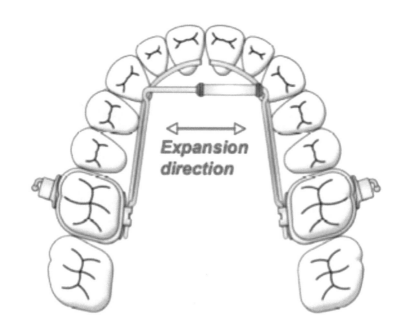

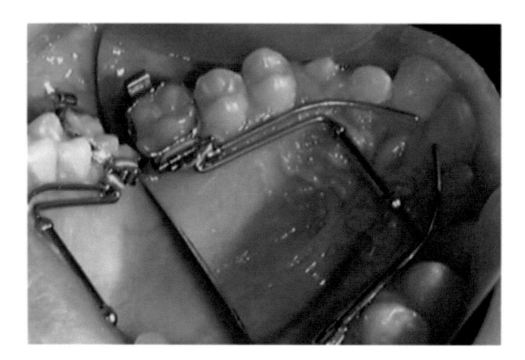

The TransForce Expander fits comfortably in the palate and has an enclosed spring that applies a gentle force to expand the arch.

TransForce Transverse Expander

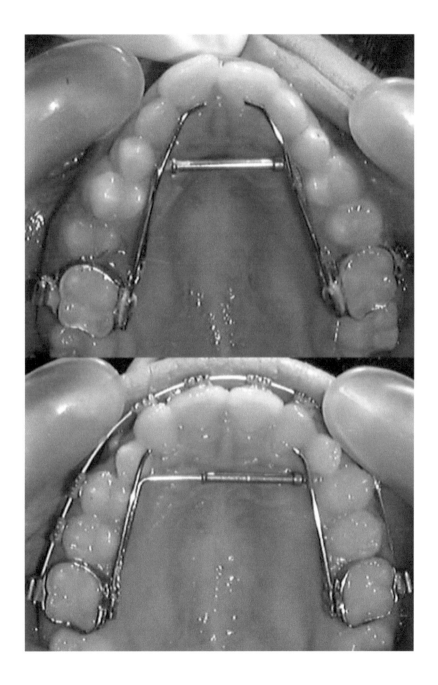

The *TransForce* appliance is used to widen the arch.

It corrects anterior crowding from early treatment through adolescence to adult therapy. TransForce appliances typically reduce the time in braces by 50%

Tony strolls into Class smiling
Hi Guys
How do you like my new braces?

What are you talking about Tony? You're not wearing braces.
I don't mean that kind of 'braces' STAR.   Look at my teeth!
You still ain't wearing no braces Dude. Who are you kidding?

Look I'll show you. Tony opens his mouth and puts his head back. it's one of these new TransForce deals. It's invisible. It fits behind my teeth,

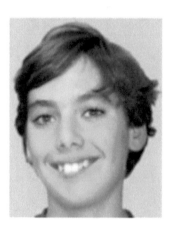 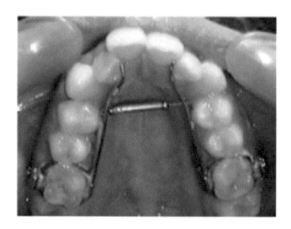

Hey Tony. That's good. That's a new one on me I haven't seen that one before. You sure do need braces to improve your image! But what does this TransForce thing do anyway?

Well my front teeth are all crooked. The Doctor calls it crowding, so he has to make my face wider so he can fit my teeth in. Ain't that just the COOLEST thing you ever heard? The swell thing is I get to wear Train Tracks for just half the time. That's what I call a real good deal!

Train Tracks ain't so bad. In fact I would go so far as to say:
It's like in that ancient Bond movie..... METAL MOUTH ......Real STRONG!
Personally I only go out with girls that have braces. After they have their braces off they are the best looking girls in Class. Forward planning pays off!

Smart choice RINGO. Maybe braces ain't so bad after all!
FOR COOL DUDES THE TIN GRIN'S THE IN THING

I Didn't Want Train Tracks

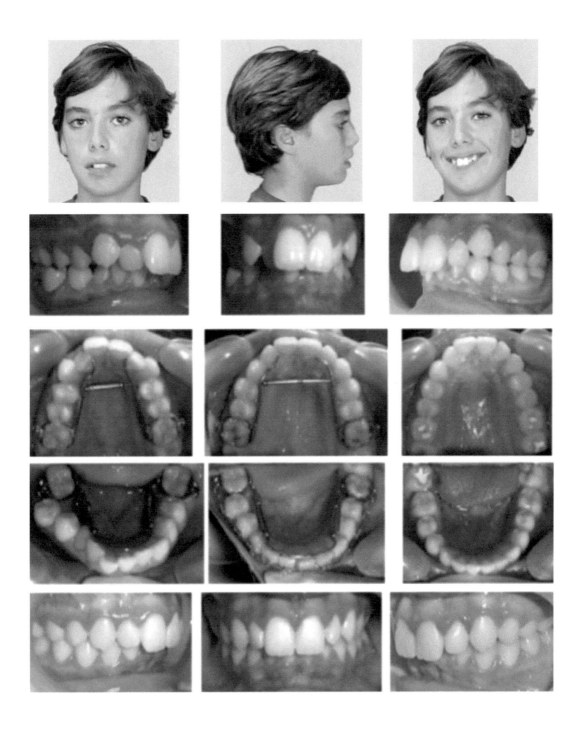

After I heard about Invisible Teen TransForce!

Invisible Teen TransForce

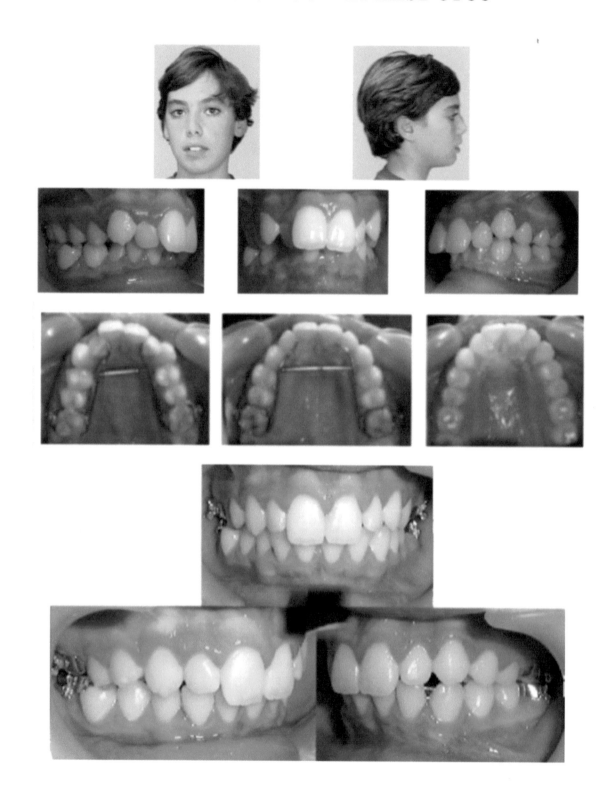

Just 4 Months Treatment !

I'm so glad I chose Teen TransForce!

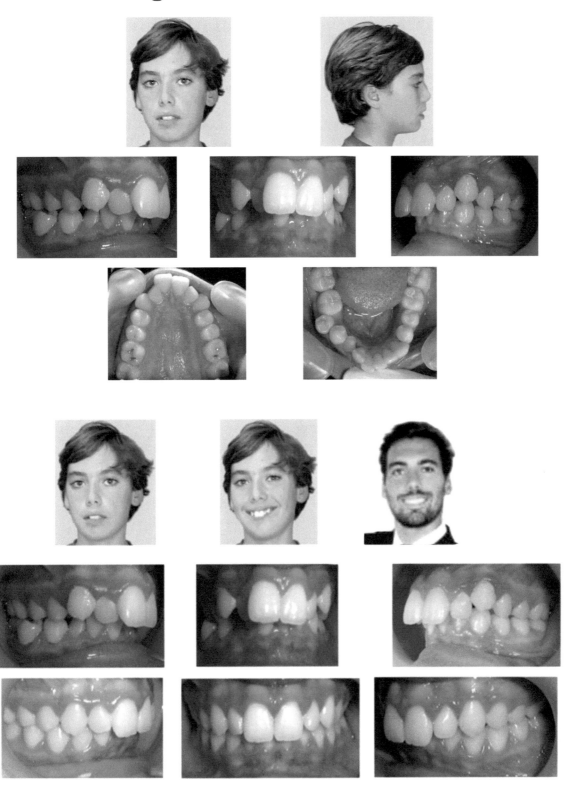

Now I can Smile with Confidence!

My teeth were crooked and outside my lips

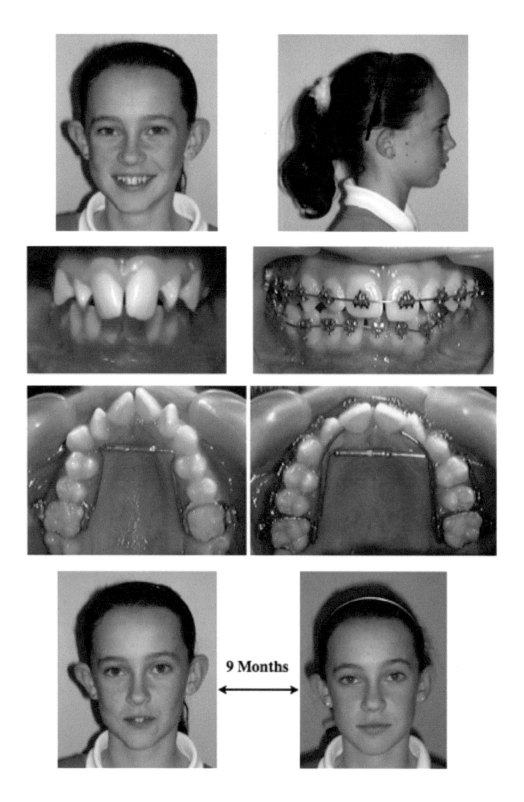

9 Months

TransForce arch development improved my face!

Transverse TransForce Expander improved my face

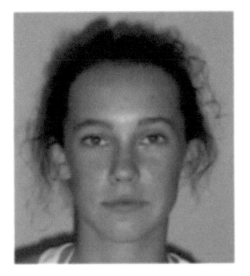 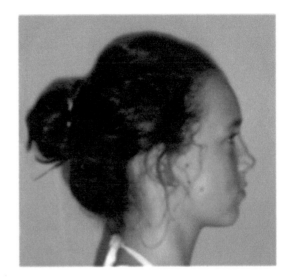

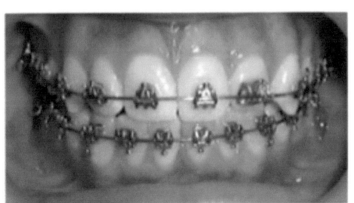

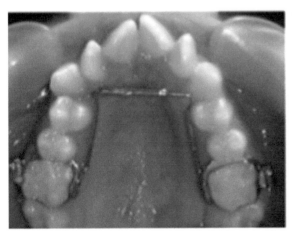 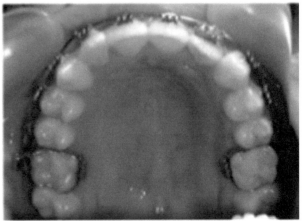

Then Train Tracks fixed my teeth

Progress With Fixed Appliances

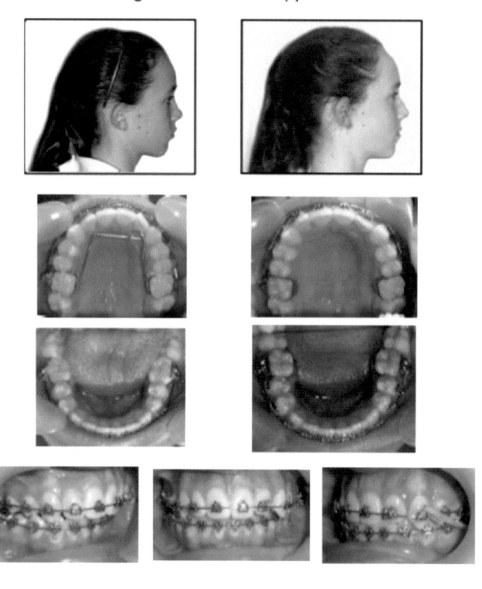

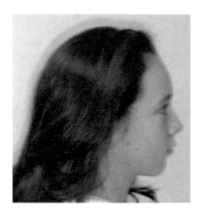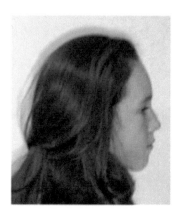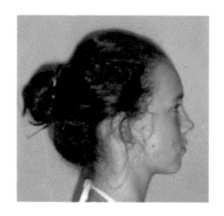

Before treatment   Mandible Postured Forward   After Twin Blocks

Twin Blocks improved my face

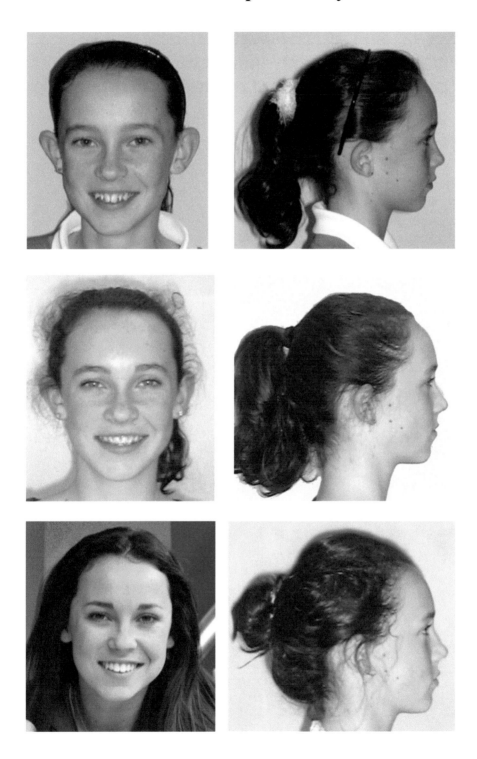

Then Train Tracks improved my smile

Q: My daughter is 8 years old. Is she too young to have braces? Do we have to wait until she is 12 ?

A: Sometimes the treatment is simpler when we start early. We can expand the arches and correct the crowding of the anterior teeth.

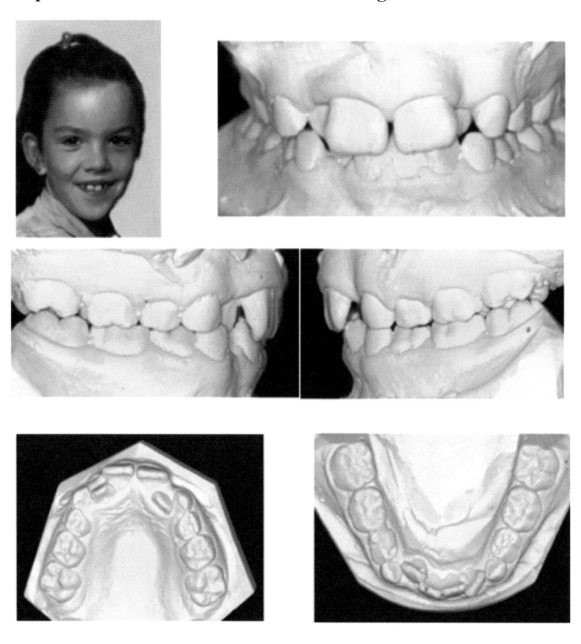

When baby teeth are still present we can often use invisible appliances that fit behind the teeth to improve the smile. Treatment is sometimes in two stages.

Train Tracks Completed My Treatment

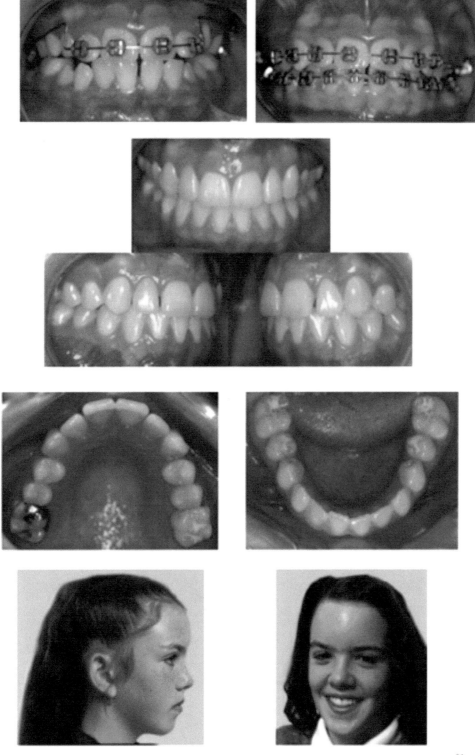

Prominent Canines Spoil Your Smile

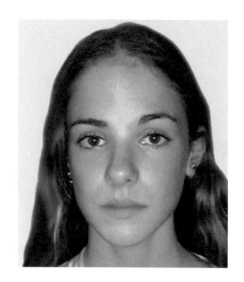
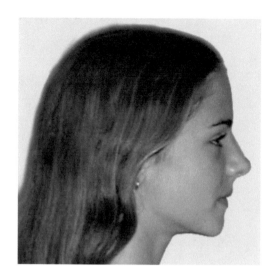
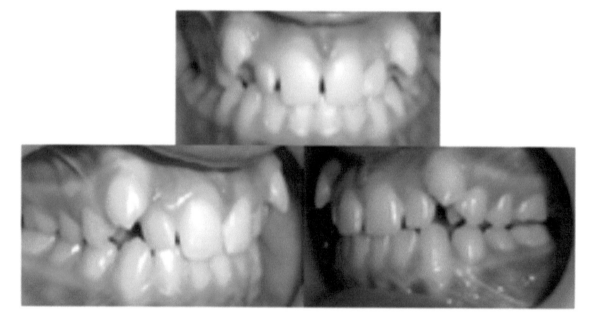
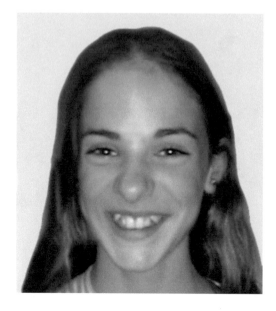

TransForce expansion to correct arch form

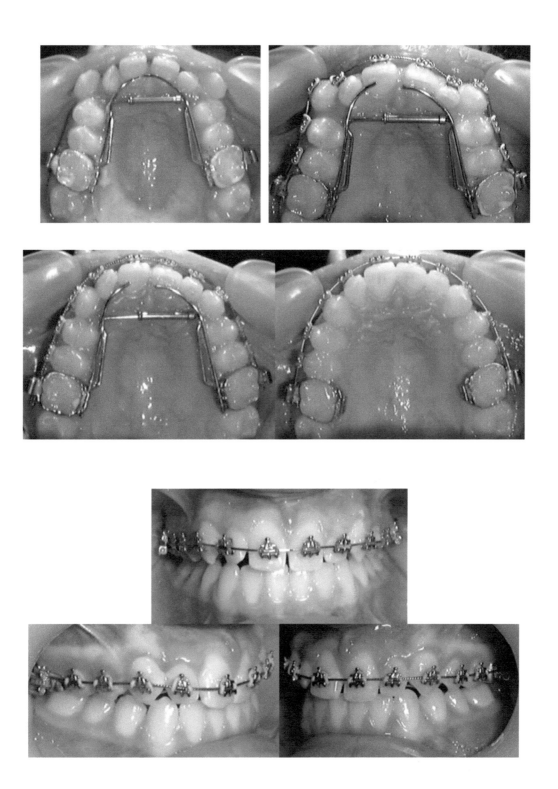

Train Tracks to complete treatment

Before & After Treatment

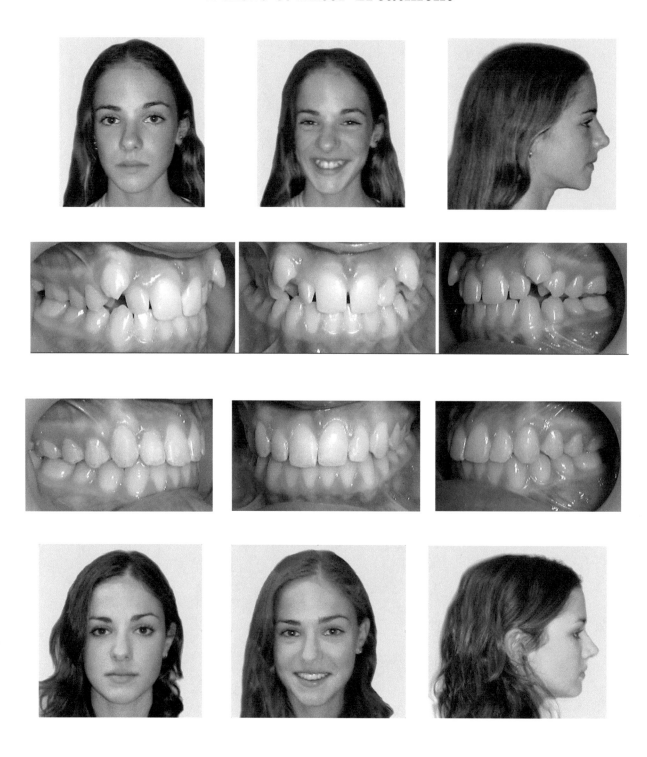

Two Years Later

A Beautiful Face & Confident Smile

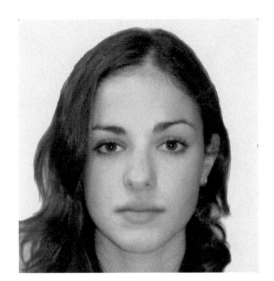 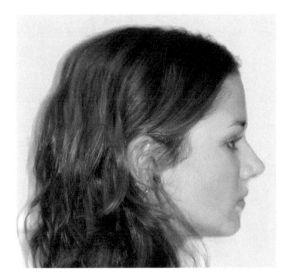

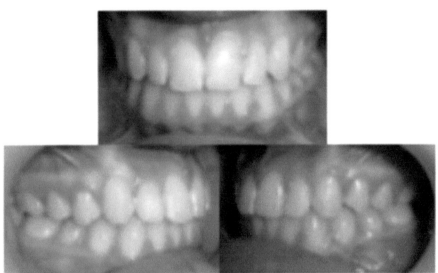

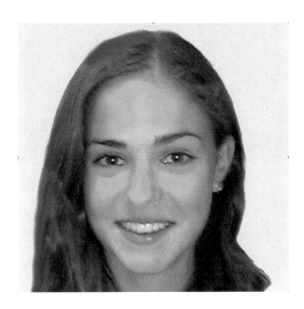

My front teeth were crooked when I was 8

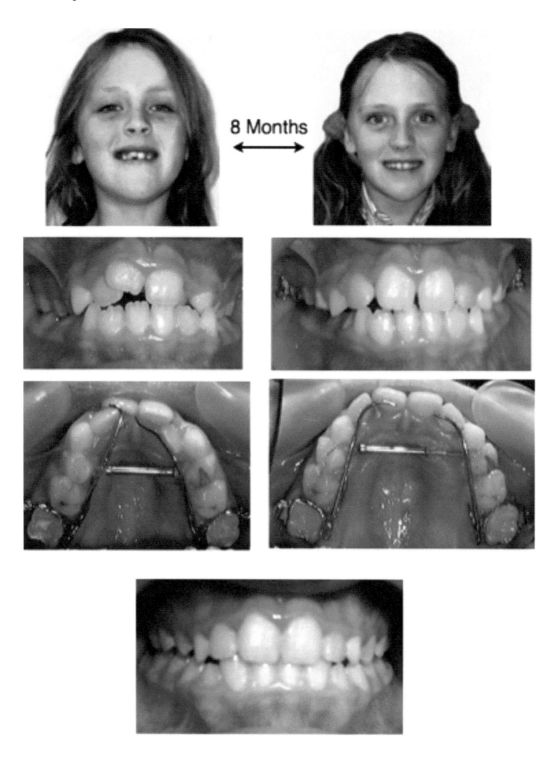

8 Months

Invisible TransForce Appliances
**Correct severe crowding of the upper incisors.
2 years later the teeth remain straight.**

Train Tracks completed my treatment

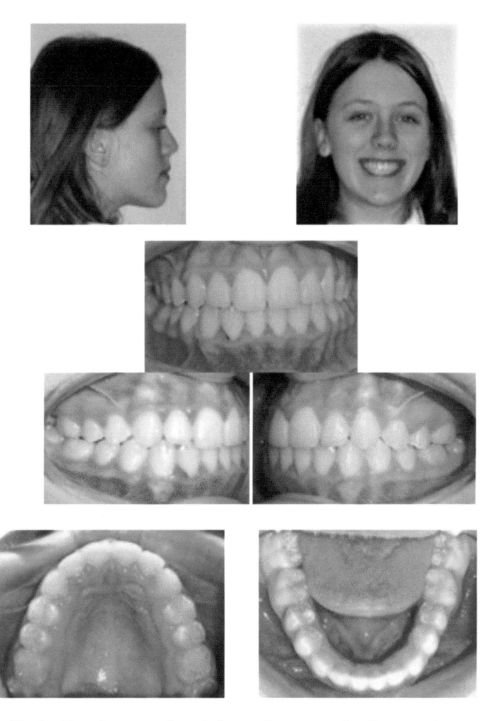

Train Tracks are fitted for a few months 3 years later to complete treatment. Early treatment may avoid extractions and *Train Tracks* are worn for a shorter time if crowding is corrected at an earlier stage.

Adults Love Invisible Braces!

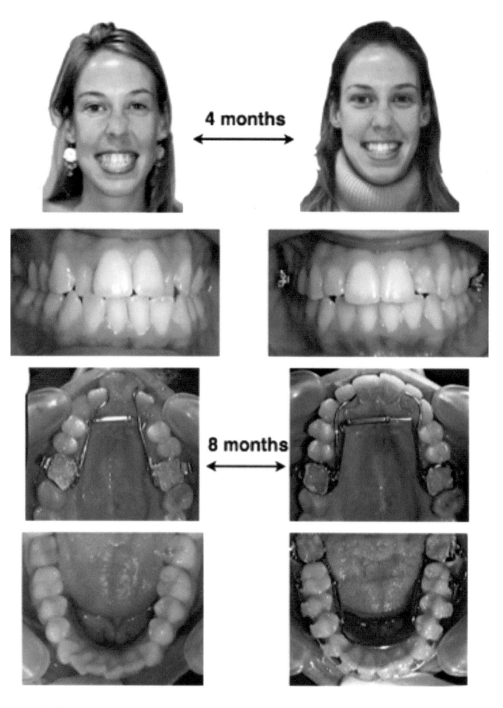

4 months

8 months

This young adult was treated with *TransForce* appliances to correct irregular anterior teeth. She enjoyed having invisible appliances for 11 months while her smile improved before proceeding to a short period with aesthetic brackets to complete treatment.

Aesthetic Brackets Completed My Treatment

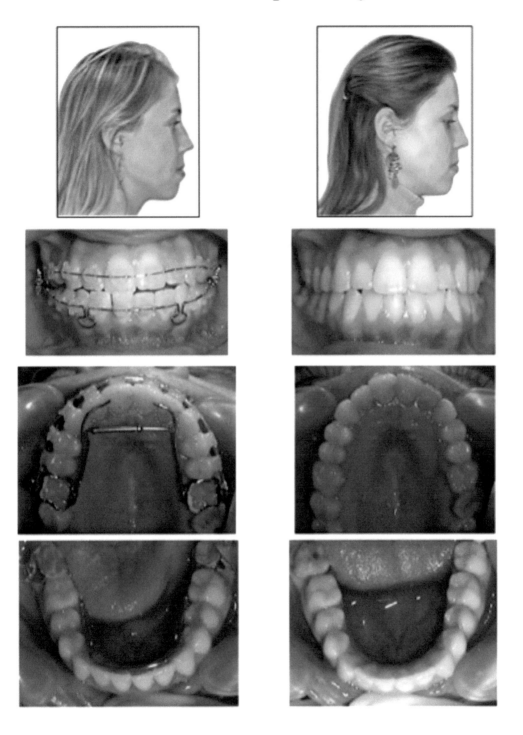

Invisible TransForce Appliances
Simplify treatment using light forces for arch development.
The time in fixed appliances is reduced by 50% followed by
invisible retainers.

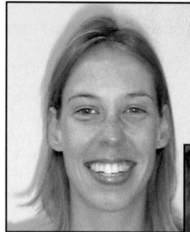

Adults Love Invisible Appliances!

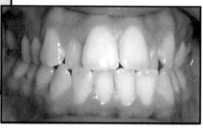

October 2004 - START   **June 2005**   **February 2006**

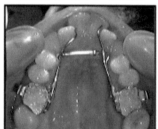
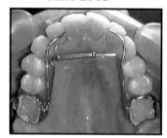
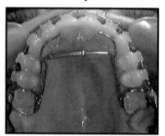

Invisible TransForce Orthodontics

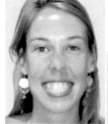

Cosmetic Appliances

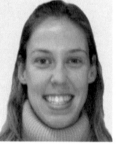

4 Months

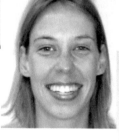

11 Months

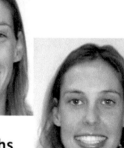

Adult Therapy   **18 Months**

Q: My teeth are straight now so why do I have to wear a retainer?
A: Retention is a very important part of orthodontic treatment. Immediately after treatment teeth would tend to go back towards their original position unless they are held securely in place by a retainer.

Removable Retainers

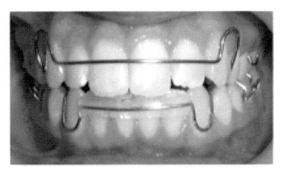

Invisible Retainers

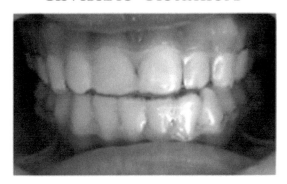

Fixed Retainers

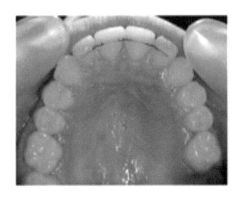 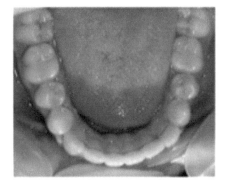

Whether your retainer is removable or fixed you must wear it exactly as instructed. Your teeth may relapse if you lose it or stop wearing it because it came off. The cost and effort of your treatment would be wasted.

It is important to wear your retainer to keep that brilliant smile.

Twin Blocks Changed My Life!

I live in India and I was so unhappy with my appearance. I was constantly teased at school and now I feel like a different person. Twin Blocks changed my life in one year and gave me confidence.

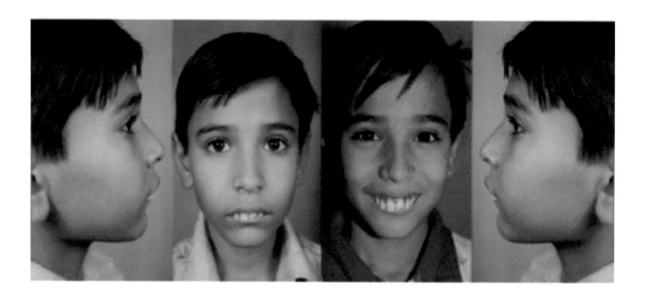

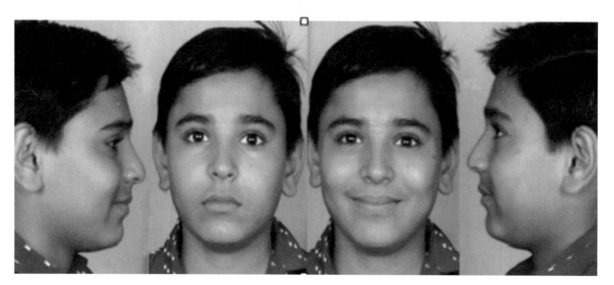

Twin Blocks are used in every country in the world for children with severe malocclusions. This treatment corrects the jaw relationship and can improve prospects for patients for the rest of their lives.
I am so glad I had Twin Blocks instead of surgery!

New Design for Invisible Twin Blocks

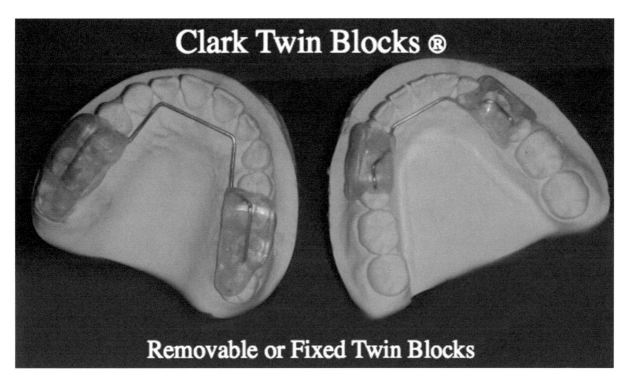

Clark Twin Blocks ®

Removable or Fixed Twin Blocks

Preformed Occclusal Blocks

Preformed Lingual Wires

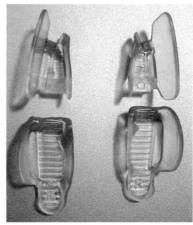

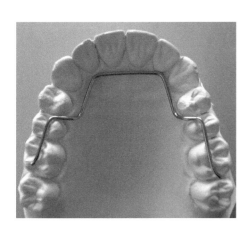

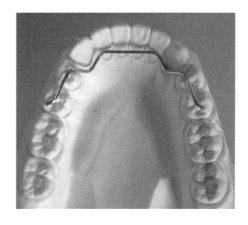

Removable or Fixed
Delivered Ready To Fit

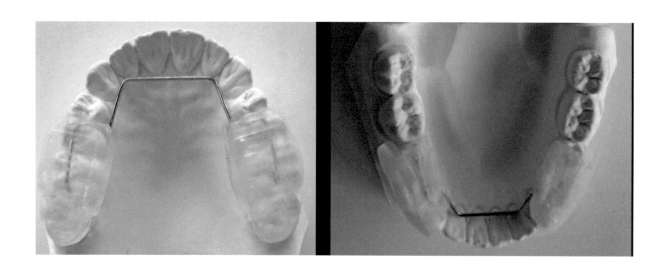

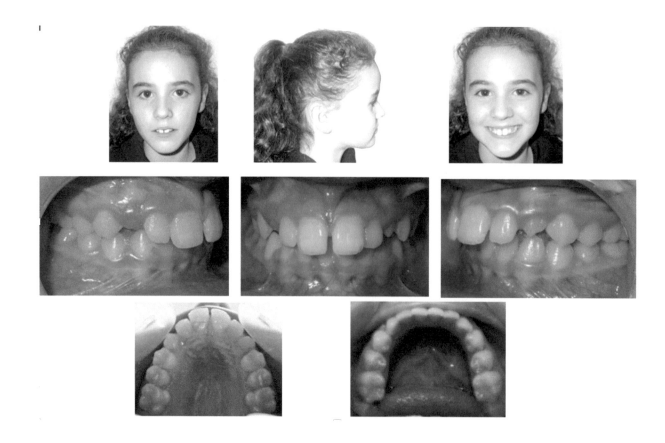

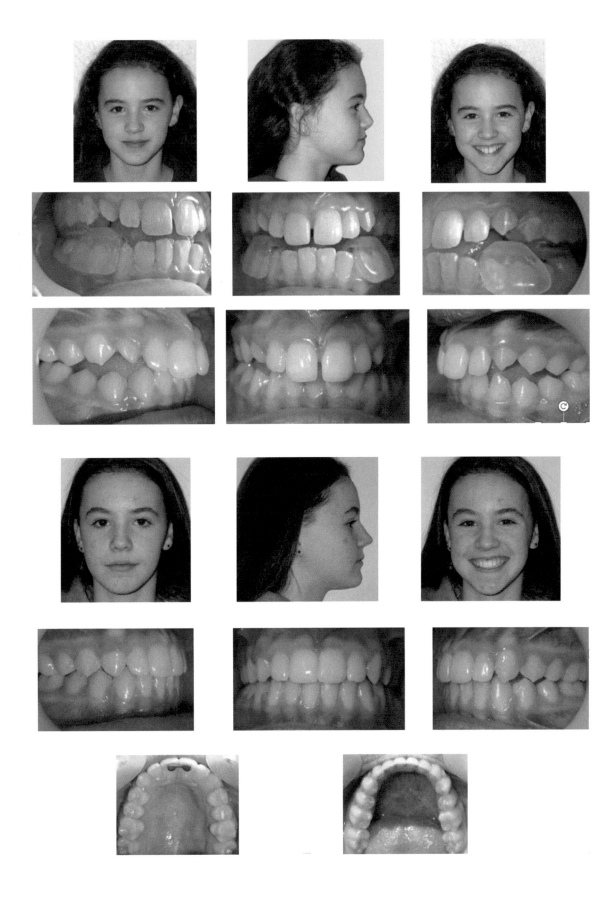

Combine Fixed & Functional Therapy

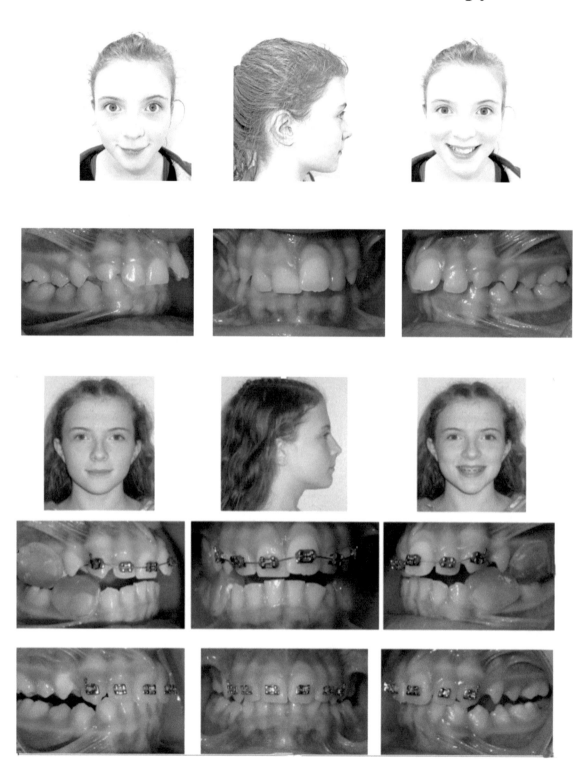

Brackets Added <u>321/123</u>

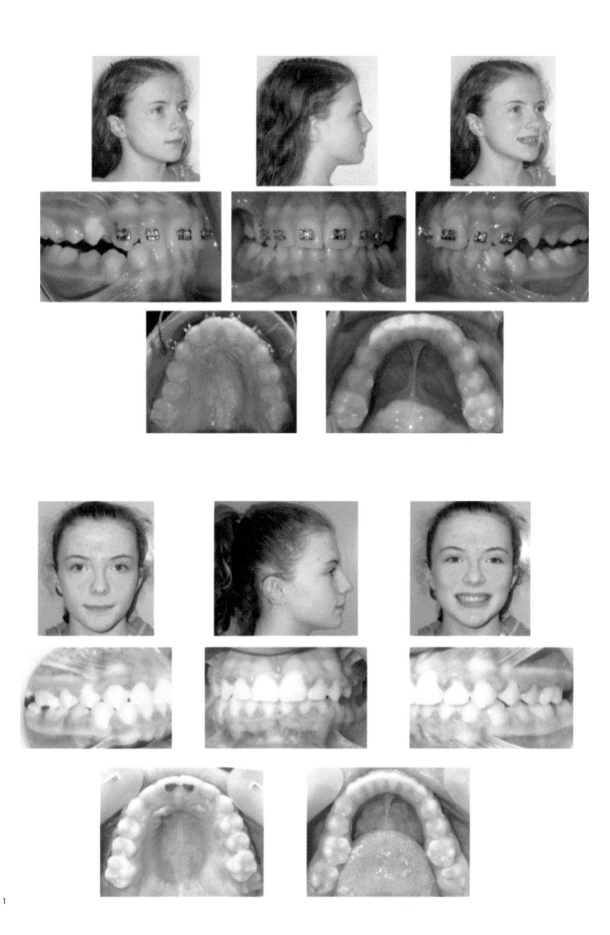

BRACES ARE COOL !!!

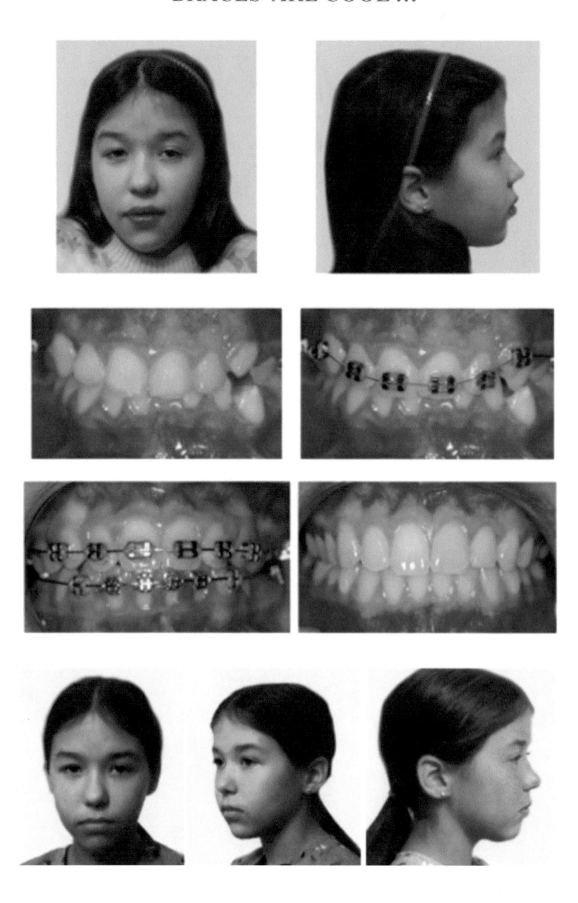

Treat Yourself to a Brilliant Smile!

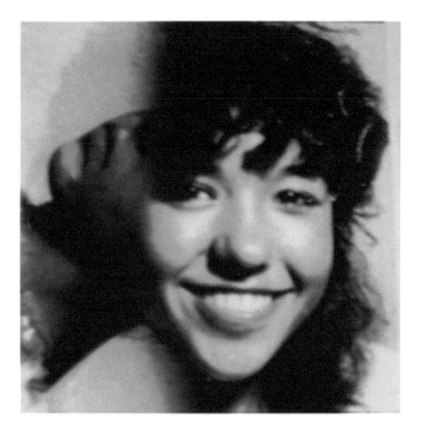

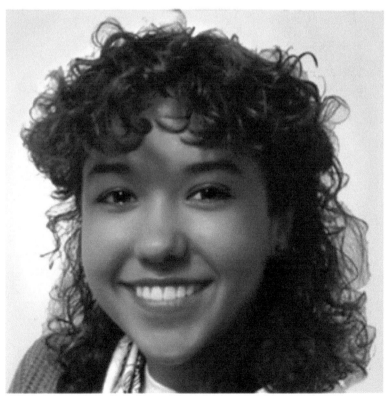

Orthodontics Can Change Your Life!

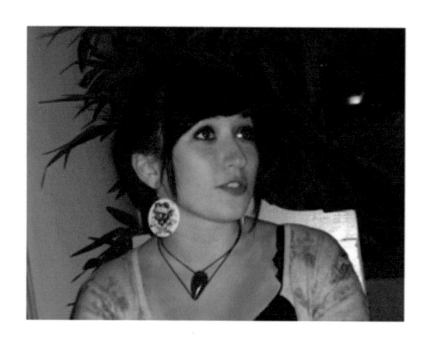

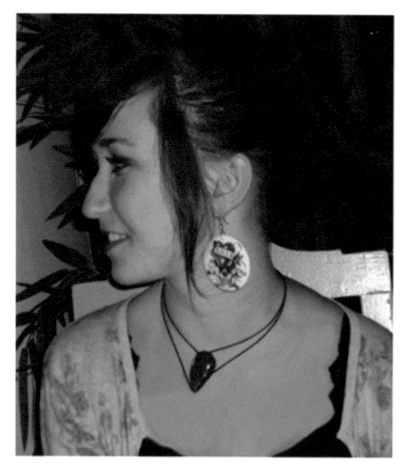

I HOPE YOU WILL DEVELOP A BRILLIANT SMILE!

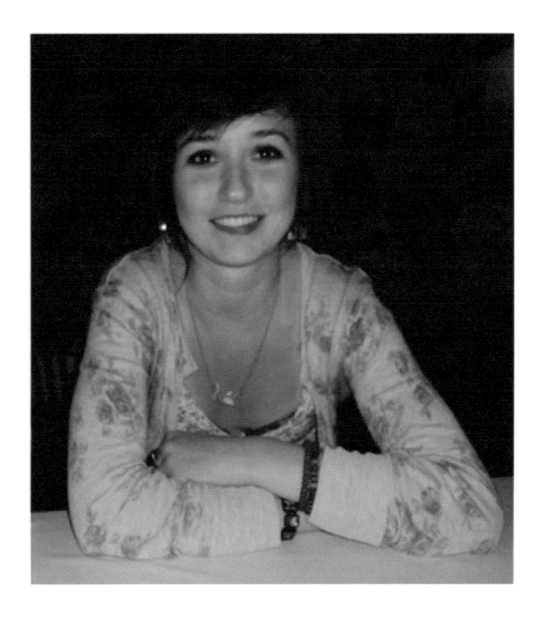

I have enjoyed talking to you and trying to help you understand why braces are brilliant, Your teeth are important in many ways. A confident smile always makes a good impression and allows you to communicate better. It improves your self image and that is a great asset in life. That is one of the rewards of orthodontic treatment. It can change your personality and improve your life as you grow up and mature.

Bon Appetit!

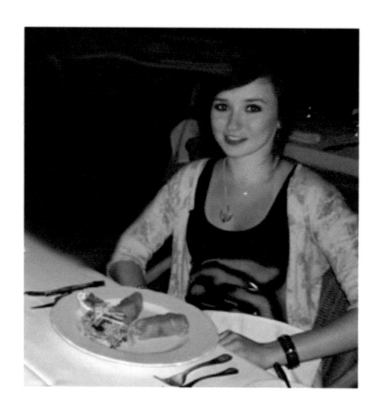

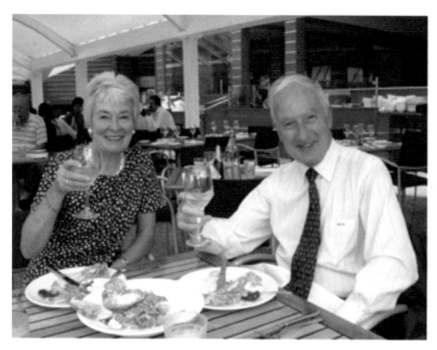

Cheers!

**Look after your teeth
You need them for the rest of your life!**

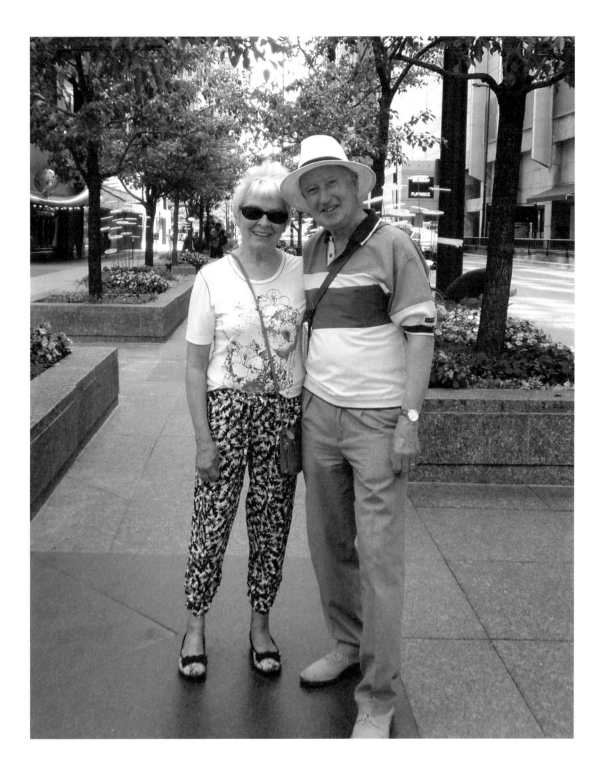

Keep Smiling!

Acknowledgements

Special thanks to Rebecca, my grand daughter, for agreeing to talk to you about Faces and Braces. and to my wife, Sheila, for proof reading and keeping me right all the time! What would I do without her?

Thanks to my son Alastair for permission to use his brilliant painting of a mask when he was 15 years old. I have used it for many years to illustrate the difference between orthodontics and dentofacial orthopaedics.

Frank Dingwall has supported me for 20 years in teaching me the finer points of computer presentation. I am indebted to Frank for his technical expertise in guiding me through the process of desktop publishing to prepare this book.

Thanks to Dr Dillip Patel and his patient from India for permission to use his treatment records to illustrate the benefits of Twin Block therapy in dentofacial orthopaedic treatment of severe malocclusion.

Although that description may sound complicated, patients worldwide have discovered that they can change their faces and develop brilliant smiles by following instructions and wearing comfortable appliances.

Whatever type of appliance you wear I wish you well in your orthodontic treatment and hope you go through life with a brilliant smile.

DEDICATION:

This book is dedicated to my patients. Without their good cooperation I could not have achieved anything. I thank them for their permission to use their records in the teaching of orthodontics. It was a pleasure and a privilege to observe them maturing as they completed their treatment and developed attractive and confident smiles.

William J. Clark

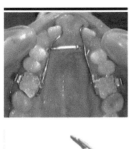
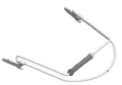
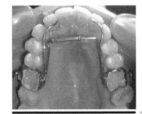
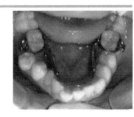

Invisible
TransForce Orthodontics

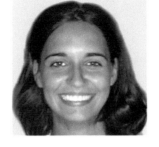

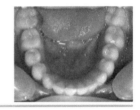

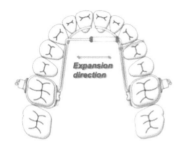
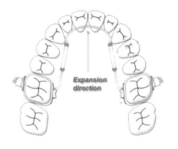

TransForm Your Smile

William J. Clark
B.D.S.,D.D.O.,D.D.Sc.,F.D.S.R.C.S. Eng

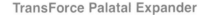

TransForce Palatal Expander   **TransForce Sagittal Expander**

This e-book on TransForce Orthodontics introduces an exciting development in interceptive orthodontics using invisble TransForce lingual appliances for arch development. Transverse and Sagittal appliances are pre-activated with enclosed nickel titanium springs to deliver light physiological forces to correct arch form from the lingual aspect.

This versatile technique has wide application in all classes of malocclusion from mixed dentition through teenage years and adolescence to adult therapy. Rapid correction without applying excessive forces is an extremeely efficient protocol to simplify correction of severe malocclusion in first phase interceptive treatment. They represent a stand alone method for correction of some malocclusions or alternatively may be followed by fixed appliances to detail the occlusion. The time required in bonded appliances is typically reduced by 50%.

TransForce Orthodontics is an excellent pre-aligner technique, which extends the range of malocclusions that may be treated with invisible appliances. This technique is more effective in producing rapid changes to simplify correction of a wide range of malocclusions prior to finishing with aligners or fixed appliances.

This book is highly recommended as it represents a revolution in interceptive orthodontics.

Find more information on www.transforceorthodontics.com

Printed in the United States
By Bookmasters